SpringerBriefs in Public Health

SpringerBriefs in Child Health

Series Editor
Angelo P. Giardino
Department of Pediatrics
Spencer Fox Eccles School of Medicine
University of Utah
Salt Lake City, UT, USA

SpringerBriefs in Child Health present concise summaries of cutting-edge research and practical applications from the fields of child and adolescent health. This book series is designed to target children's health issues from birth through adolescence, from both a policy and practice perspective. Each subject in the series will be written by a specialist in that area. Their expertise will offer evaluation of the special health issues that would be of value to any health care provider. The authors all practice at nationally recognized children's hospitals and have done extensive research in their respective areas. The "template" for the series will be in three sections: • "Snapshot from the Field" will address current practice and policy • "Implications for Policy and Practice" will deal with the emerging science and best practices related to cutting edge work going on in the field • "Looking Ahead" will look forward towards anticipated changes, recommendations and strategies to achieve the best for children and families. Featuring compact volumes of 55 to 125 pages, the series covers a range of content from professional to academic. Possible volumes in the series may consist of timely reports of state-of-the art analytical techniques, reports from the field, snapshots of hot and/or emerging topics, elaborated theses, literature reviews, and in-depth case studies. Both solicited and unsolicited manuscripts are considered for publication in this series. Briefs are published as part of Springer's eBook collection, with millions of users worldwide. In addition, Briefs are available for individual print and electronic purchase. Briefs are characterized by fast, global electronic dissemination, standard publishing contracts, easy-to-use manuscript preparation and formatting guidelines, and expedited production schedules. We aim for publication 8-12 weeks after acceptance.

Nancy Murphy • Justin C. Alvey •
Jennifer Brinton • Natalie Heyrend Darro •
Jason Fox • E. Avery Hill • Kathleen Irby •
Andrew Robertson • Laura Smals-Murphy

Healthcare Delivery for Children with Medical Complexity

The State of the Art and Future Directions

With Contribution by Stefanie Ames

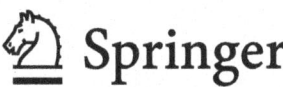

Nancy Murphy
Department of Pediatrics, Division of Pediatric
Complex Care, Spencer Fox Eccles
School of Medicine, University of Utah
Salt Lake City, UT, USA

Jennifer Brinton
Department of Pediatrics, Division
of Pediatric Complex Care
Spencer Fox Eccles School of Medicine,
University of Utah
Salt Lake City, UT, USA

Jason Fox
Department of Pediatrics,
Clinical Revenue Integrity
Spencer Fox Eccles School of Medicine,
University of Utah
Salt Lake City, UT, USA

Kathleen Irby
Department of Pediatrics, Division of Pediatric
Complex Care, Spencer Fox Eccles School of
Medicine, University of Utah
Salt Lake City, UT, USA

Laura Smals-Murphy
Department of Pediatrics, Division
of Pediatric Complex Care
Spencer Fox Eccles School of Medicine,
University of Utah
Salt Lake City, UT, USA

Justin C. Alvey
Department of Pediatrics, Division
of General Pediatrics
Spencer Fox Eccles School of Medicine,
University of Utah
Salt Lake City, UT, USA

Natalie Heyrend Darro
Department of Pediatrics, Division
of Pediatric Complex Care
Spencer Fox Eccles School of Medicine,
University of Utah
Salt Lake City, UT, USA

E. Avery Hill
Department of Pediatrics, Division
of Pediatric Complex Care
Spencer Fox Eccles School of Medicine,
University of Utah
Salt Lake City, UT, USA

Andrew Robertson
Department of Pediatrics, Division
of Pediatric Complex Care
Spencer Fox Eccles School of Medicine,
University of Utah
Salt Lake City, UT, USA

ISSN 2192-3698　　　　　　　　ISSN 2192-3701　(electronic)
SpringerBriefs in Public Health
ISSN 2625-2872　　　　　　　　ISSN 2625-2880　(electronic)
SpringerBriefs in Child Health
ISBN 978-3-031-93346-2　　　　ISBN 978-3-031-93347-9　(eBook)
https://doi.org/10.1007/978-3-031-93347-9

© The Editor(s) (if applicable) and The Author(s), under exclusive license to Springer Nature Switzerland AG 2025

This work is subject to copyright. All rights are solely and exclusively licensed by the Publisher, whether the whole or part of the material is concerned, specifically the rights of translation, reprinting, reuse of illustrations, recitation, broadcasting, reproduction on microfilms or in any other physical way, and transmission or information storage and retrieval, electronic adaptation, computer software, or by similar or dissimilar methodology now known or hereafter developed.
The use of general descriptive names, registered names, trademarks, service marks, etc. in this publication does not imply, even in the absence of a specific statement, that such names are exempt from the relevant protective laws and regulations and therefore free for general use.
The publisher, the authors and the editors are safe to assume that the advice and information in this book are believed to be true and accurate at the date of publication. Neither the publisher nor the authors or the editors give a warranty, expressed or implied, with respect to the material contained herein or for any errors or omissions that may have been made. The publisher remains neutral with regard to jurisdictional claims in published maps and institutional affiliations.

This Springer imprint is published by the registered company Springer Nature Switzerland AG
The registered company address is: Gewerbestrasse 11, 6330 Cham, Switzerland

If disposing of this product, please recycle the paper.

Foreword

The health care of children with medical complexity (CMC), a small but increasingly important population of children, is and has been a tremendous challenge for the US healthcare system. Historically, the care and management of chronic conditions has been mainly adult-focused, and the health care of children has been the subject of relatively little attention on the part of payers and policymakers. Fortunately, the pediatric sector (especially children's hospitals) and the child health services research community has gradually been paying much more attention to CMC over the last 50 years. CMC represent an increasing share of work in this sector by virtue of their increased survival rates, their overall increasing complexity, and possibly increased prevalence in the population over time. CMC require support from multiple sectors: health care (including mental and behavioral health), community resources, education, and others, and it is essential that these supports be well coordinated to ensure their effectiveness and efficiency. This monograph is one of the first to address these tough issues, covering several major aspects of the care of CMC from a systems perspective along with practical applications based on the authors' experience.

Though definitions vary, most agree that the most medically complex children comprise between 1% and 1.5% of the US child population, or around 1 million children. CMC are an important population not only because of their disproportionate share of healthcare expenditures and provider work, but because their care is uniquely difficult. Their needs include not only care from the "traditional" healthcare sector of primary and specialty medical care, but also multiple habilitative therapies, special education, and nursing and other services provided at home. Health-related social needs in the CMC population are even more prevalent than in the non-CMC population, especially when CMC from higher socioeconomic status families are compared with non-CMC. None of these systems are well designed to provide integrated care, leaving many families feeling like they are quite alone in pursuing resources that meet their child's specific needs. Many providers within each sector feel uncomfortable providing care for CMC, compounding problems with access to services.

One bright spot in the care of CMC over the last 25–30 years has been the emergence of complex care programs, mostly affiliated with children's hospitals. These programs are described in detail in this monograph. They may have inpatient and/or outpatient components, and models vary from a consultative model, where children are seen as with most subspecialties to aid in diagnostic and management plans, to a complete medical home model, where children receive comprehensive primary care and may even be cared for by the same teams when they are admitted to hospital. Typically, they include several disciplines such as nutrition and have care coordination expertise and capacity that few other models of care have. These programs are favored highly by families and much appreciated by community providers. Some have been shown to decrease avoidable emergency department visits and hospitalizations and potentially other costs to the system, although their own cost to run is considerable due to the large team involved, and they cannot generate positive revenue on their own. While these programs are tremendously valuable for the children and families they serve, capacity is limited, and they typically serve a few hundred to a couple of thousand patients at most. Given the sheer number of CMC in the USA and access problems for children not within easy reach of academic medical centers, it is clear that complex care programs cannot be the only model of care for CMC. Engagement and support of community providers as team members, including primary care practices and other non-academically based resources, is essential to provide care for all CMC.

What would such support look like? It may include seamless communication; differing degrees of consultation or co-management between community sites and complex care programs, including consultation from nutrition, nursing, and care coordination services; telephone support; synchronous and/or asynchronous telehealth visits, including the potential for joint visits between the complex care program and community site; and/or other supports. Currently, neither delivery nor payment systems are set up to enable, much less incentivize, this hard work. Services have developed their own "silos" of care, with no incentives to collaborate. Payment is still inadequate for the time and expertise needed, as well as being largely in fee-for-service structures despite more than 20 years of recognition that such models cannot adequately fund team-based care for CMC. If comprehensive, team-based care for CMC is to be viable, both system and payment structures must change to make caring for CMC not just possible but attractive.

For the same reasons, while "complexology" has emerged as a new potential pediatric subspecialty, it is not an innovation that will help the care of CMC in any dramatic fashion by itself. Decades of experience and data on access to care, workforce, and payment, as discussed in the 2023 National Academies of Sciences, Engineering, and Medicine (NASEM) consensus study report on the pediatric subspecialty workforce, raise significant concerns about this approach. Emerging pediatric subspecialties, whose work is primarily outpatient-focused and cognitively based, with their attendant training and certification requirements, are having increasing difficulty attracting pediatricians and present significant barriers to workforce development and subsequent access to care. However, new curricula around team care for CMC are a huge bright spot for the field and can and should be promoted within residency training. With this enhanced knowledge and the opportunity to use it, general pediatricians can be well equipped to care for the great majority of CMC. It is easy to imagine that interested, well-trained community general pediatricians and their teams could work together with complex care specialists to achieve similar outcomes as those experienced within complex care programs. Again, however, the current system and payment structures that incentivize neither team care nor coordination of services discourage their active participation in leading care teams.

Finally, and perhaps most importantly, partnerships on a deep level between professionals and families of CMC are essential to make processes of care work. Families know their children and the ecosystem and community within which they live, learn, and play best. Even the best electronic health record system cannot capture the important nuances of health and health care that families can encounter during their child's journey. Collaborative learning and support among families and care team members brings joy to the often difficult care process, and promoting and celebrating that joy can attract others to this incredibly fulfilling work. I am hopeful that this monograph will help to spark interest and serve as a roadmap for those interested in joining our big team.

Children's Hospital Colorado Christopher Stille
Aurora, CO, USA

Contents

1 Children with Medical Complexity: Who They Are and Why Caring for Them Matters 1
   Introduction. 1
   Defining Children with Medical Complexity 1
   Public Health and Children with Medical Complexity 3
   Emergence of Complex Care Programs for Children with Medical Complexity 4
   International Classification of Function and the "F Words" 5
   The Right to Education.. 6
   The Collaborative Improvement and Innovation Network to Advance Care for Children with Medical Complexity 7
   Looking Forward. 7
   References. 8

2 The Specialty and Scope of Complex Care Pediatrics 11
   Introduction. 11
   Who Are Complex Care Pediatricians? 12
   Complex Care Education and Training. 12
   Emergence of Complex Care Programs: A Potpourri of Models and Services 13
      The Medical Home vs. the Medical Neighborhood 14
      Systems/Models of Service. 14
   Multidisciplinary Collaborations for Children with Medical Complexity: A Conglomeration of Needs. 16
      Shared Decision Making for Children with Medical Complexity 16
      Children with Dependence on Home Mechanical Ventilation: Tracheostomy/Ventilator Program 18
      Complex Surgeries in Children with Medical Complexity. 19
      The Intersections of Complex Care and Palliative Care 21

	Coordination of Care and Integration with Community Systems.......	23
	Definitions and Framework of Care Coordination: The How's and The Why's	23
	The Benefits of Care Coordination Within Practices and Integration with Community Resources: The Who's and the What's..	24
	Systems for Transitions to Adulthood for Children with Medical Complexity.......................................	27
	Transition Gaps, Barriers, and Solutions	31
	References...	33
3	**Community and Family Partnerships**...........................	39
	Social Determinants of Health and Children with Medical Complexity..	39
	Impact on Siblings of Children with Medical Complexity............	40
	Future Directions	41
	Medicaid and State Waiver Programs............................	42
	Home Nursing and Families as Caregivers.......................	42
	Resiliency of Caregivers.......................................	43
	Organizational Resources for Families of Children with Medical Complexity.......................................	46
	Partnering with Families.................................	46
	References...	47
4	**Ethical Considerations in the Care of Children with Medical Complexity**...	51
	Children with Medical Complexity: Focusing on the Big Picture	51
	Promoting the Child's Best Interests.............................	52
	Decision Making with Complexity and Uncertainty	53
	What Is the Right "Dose" of Care?...........................	54
	Growth Attenuation Therapy: An Example of Shared Decision Making	55
	Complementary and Alternative Medicine	56
	Decision Making, Autonomy, and Support in the Transition to Adulthood..	57
	Children with Medical Complexity: US Disability Rights and Challenges..	61
	Ableism: A Modern-Day Issue for Children with Medical Complexity...	62
	References...	63
5	**Implications for Policy and Practice**............................	69
	Introduction...	69
	Definition of Children with Medical Complexity....................	70
	Demographics..	71
	Direct Healthcare Costs	72

	Indirect Healthcare Costs	72
	Models of Care	73
	Ambulatory	73
	Inpatient	74
	Models of Payment	76
	Chronic Care Management Programs	77
	Funds Flow Models	80
	Accountable Care Organizations	81
	Medicaid for Children with Medical Complexity	82
	Medicaid Waivers	82
	The ACE Kids Act	83
	Toward Bridging the Quality Chasm	85
	References	86
6	**Looking Ahead: Children with Medical Complexity and Public Health, Workforce Training, and Advocacy**	**91**
	A Healthcare System Call to Action	91
	A Well-Prepared Pediatric Workforce	92
	Strong and Steady Pediatric Advocacy	94
	Families as Providers, Educators, and Advocates	94
	Pediatricians as Legislative Advocates	95
	Advocacy with Payers, Policy Makers, and Community Stakeholders	96
	Summary and Future Directions	96
	References	97
Index		**99**

About the Authors and Contributor

About the Authors

Nancy Murphy, MD, FAAP, FAAPMR, is Professor of Pediatrics, Adjunct Professor of Physical Medicine & Rehabilitation, and Chief of the Division of Pediatric Complex Care at the University of Utah Department of Pediatrics. She focuses her clinical and academic efforts on optimizing function, quality of life, participation, and wellness for children with complex medical conditions and disabilities and their families. Dr. Murphy uniquely blends her expertise as a pediatrician, a pediatric physiatrist, and an academic health leader to build and connect people and processes in team-based, interdependent systems. She is a fellow of Drexel University's Executive Leadership in Academic Medicine (ELAM 2020). She serves as the Vice Chair of Faculty Engagement and Director of Women in Pediatrics in the Department of Pediatrics. Dr. Murphy designs, implements, and sustains processes that enhance the interpersonal and professional experiences of pediatric faculty.

Justin C. Alvey, MD, FAAP, received his medical degree from Washington University School of Medicine in St. Louis, MO. He completed his pediatric residency at the University of Utah School of Medicine/Primary Children's Hospital. Dr. Alvey is an experienced general pediatrician who practiced in the community for over 15 years prior to joining the faculty at the University of Utah as Associate Professor of Pediatrics in the Division of General Pediatrics. He currently sees patients in the Comprehensive Care Program at Primary Children's Hospital and at the University of Utah Pediatric Clinic. In those settings, Dr. Alvey sees a wide range of patients of all ages and health conditions. Dr. Alvey's clinical interests include providing primary care for children with complex medical problems, ADHD, asthma, and underlying genetic, metabolic, and neurological disorders.

Jennifer Brinton, MD, FAAP, cares for children as a general pediatrician at South Davis Community Hospital Skilled Nursing Facility and Long-Term Acute Care, Neurorestorative Skilled Nursing Facility, and as a hospitalist at Primary Children's Hospital. She has a special interest in disease prevention, child advocacy, and the comprehensive care of children with special healthcare needs. She volunteers on the Utah Medicaid Advisory Committee and the Medicaid Drug Utilization Review Board and is involved in leadership for the Utah Chapter of the American Academy of Pediatrics and the Utah Medical Association, advocating for healthcare coverage for our most vulnerable children. Dr. Brinton graduated from the University of Utah School of Medicine and completed her residency in categorical pediatrics at the institution. She was a partner with Utah Valley Pediatrics (UVPEDS) in Orem, Utah, for 5 ½ years. While in practice, she participated in Utah Pediatric Partnership to Improve Healthcare Quality (UPIQ) quality improvement projects in asthma, ADHD, and medical home and applied for and was awarded a grant from the Utah Chapter of the American Lung Association for an asthma quality improvement project. She was the chair of the Quality Improvement Committee for UVPEDS her last two years in practice and served as a volunteer pediatrician at the Utah County United Way free clinic once a month for two years.

Natalie Heyrend Darro, DO, FAAP, is Assistant Professor of Pediatrics at the University of Utah School of Medicine in the Division of Pediatric Complex Care. She cares for children with medical complexity and disabilities in the Comprehensive Care Program at Primary Children's Outpatient Services as well as in the Pediatric Transitional Care Program at South Davis Community Hospital. Dr. Darro earned her medical degree from Touro University Nevada College of Osteopathic Medicine, completed her pediatric residency at the University of Nevada School of Medicine in Las Vegas, and her fellowship in pediatric critical care at the University of California San Diego at Rady Children's Hospital. She is board certified in pediatrics and pediatric critical care. She practiced for several years in a community pediatric intensive care unit prior to joining the faculty in the Comprehensive Care Program. Dr. Darro's clinical interests include providing consultative care for children with complex medical conditions and medical fragility with more specific interest in children who are recovering from traumatic brain injury, have congenital heart disease, have received transplants or are awaiting organ transplantation, and have neurodegenerative disorders and children who are dependent on medical technologies.

Jason Fox, MPA/MHA, is the Director of Clinical Revenue Integrity & Primary Care Operations for the Department of Pediatrics at the University of Utah School of Medicine. He also serves as the Division Manager for Adolescent Medicine, Complex Care, and General Pediatrics. Jason graduated from the University of Utah with master's degrees in public administration and healthcare administration. He has a background in quality improvement while working on a Patient-Centered Medical Home Demonstration Grant through the Children's Health Insurance Program Reauthorization Act (CHIPRA). He is also a graduate of, and current faculty member in, the Utah Regional Leadership Education in Neurodevelopmental and Related Disabilities (URLEND) program. Jason has a passion for embracing a quality improvement approach to increase quality and access for underserved populations while also trying to improve and increase value for all that interact in the healthcare landscape.

E. Avery Hill, DO, FAAP, first developed a passion for working with people with disabilities as a teenager volunteering at the National Ability Center in Park City, Utah. After attending medical school in Rocky Vista University College of Osteopathic Medicine in Parker, Colorado, and completing her pediatric residency at Blank Children's Hospital in Des Moines, Iowa, she became the inaugural fellow of Complex Care Pediatrics at the University of Utah. Her passions include advocacy and partnering with families to provide the best care possible to children with medical complexity. When she is not in clinic, Avery can be found skiing or hiking with her golden retriever.

Kathleen Irby, MD, is Assistant Professor of Internal Medicine and Pediatrics at the University of Utah. After graduating from medical school at Nebraska Medicine, she completed an internal medicine-pediatrics residency at the University of Utah followed by fellowships in adult developmental medicine at the Baylor College of Medicine and hospice and palliative medicine at the University of Utah. She now splits her clinical time between the Divisions of Pediatric Complex Care at Primary Children's Hospital and Palliative Medicine at the University of Utah, where she is working to develop an adult medical home for patients with intellectual and developmental disabilities.

Andrew Robertson, PA-C, received his Master of Medical Science in Physician Assistant Studies from Midwestern University in Glendale, Arizona. Prior to that, he earned a degree in Exercise and Sports Science from the University of Utah. Andy enjoys his work on the Comprehensive Care team where he is able to collaborate with many providers in taking care of children with medical complexity. He aspires to teach the next generation of physician assistants.

Laura Smals-Murphy, MD, is Associate Professor of Pediatrics at the University of Utah in the Division of Pediatric Complex Care. She joined the University of Utah in July 2023. Previously she had been in Pennsylvania for over 20 years, caring for children with medical complexity in two primary care medical homes that she was instrumental in creating—one at St. Christopher's Hospital for Children in Philadelphia and one at Penn State Children's Hospital in Hershey, PA. She has leadership experience in the education of medical students and residents and has a passion for teaching the next generation the skills of caring for children with medical complexity in multiple settings.

About the Contributor

Stefanie Ames, MD, MS, received her medical degree from the Southern Illinois University School of Medicine, completed her Pediatric residency at Primary Children's Hospital, and her Critical Care Fellowship at Children's Hospital of Pittsburgh. Dr. Ames is board certified in Pediatrics and Pediatric Critical Care. She is currently Associate Professor of Pediatrics at the University of Utah, where she cares for children with complex conditions, critical illness, and injury in the Pediatric Intensive Care Unit. Her research interests focus on improving care for children with special healthcare needs including understanding and addressing ableism in pediatric health care.

Chapter 1
Children with Medical Complexity: Who They Are and Why Caring for Them Matters

Introduction

Children with medical complexity (CMC) are a growing population of children who have multiple complex chronic health conditions, functional limitations, and technology dependencies. CMC require significant and specialized health services and are among the highest utilizers of pediatric healthcare resources. This small yet important pediatric population has a great impact on pediatric healthcare systems, their families, and their communities. CMC are a subgroup of children and youth with special healthcare needs (CYSHCN), defined as children who "have or are at increased risk for a chronic physical, developmental, behavioral, or emotional condition and who require health and related services of a type or amount beyond that required by children generally" (McPherson et al., 1998). CYSHCN account for 13–18% of the US pediatric population (Cohen et al., 2011), whereas CMC account for 1% of all US children (Kuo et al., 2016). Advances in medical care and community-based services for CMC support this growing population of children who would have historically succumbed to their life limiting conditions. The population of CMC is rapidly growing, with many of these children successfully transitioning into adulthood (Kuo et al., 2011).

Defining Children with Medical Complexity

Children with medical complexity have been described by several frameworks (Feudtner et al., 2014; Simon et al., 2018; Cohen et al., 2011), yet the heterogeneity of this population has precluded a single, widely implemented classification system. In general, CMC are defined as children with at least three organ systems affected, significant functional limitations, technology dependencies, and high healthcare resource utilization. A child with anoxic encephalopathy, epilepsy, spastic quadriplegic cerebral palsy, neuromuscular scoliosis, gastrostomy tube dependency, and multiple functional limitations is a CMC. So too are infants born with extreme prematurity, severe bronchopulmonary dysplasia requiring tracheostomies and/or home ventilators, dysphagia with gastrostomy tube dependencies, and vision and hearing impairments. Children with metabolic, neuromuscular, and/or genetic disorders that are associated with increasing complexity and decreasing function as they age are also CMC. All these children with widely varying diagnoses meet the definition of CMC, with unifying features of multi-system conditions, technology dependencies, and functional limitations. Table 1.1 provides further examples of CMC.

> **In Our Experience**
> While there has been a lot of work done to create an objective definition of medical complexity, each of the models falls short—either leaving complex patients excluded or including patients that are not truly complex. An experienced complex care provider can identify medically complex children, and complex care programs need to have the ability to use that clinical instinct to override defined criteria when appropriate.

CMC need interdisciplinary teams of providers, including primary care pediatricians, medical and surgical subspecialists, home health nurses, rehabilitation providers (physical therapists, speech/language pathologists, occupational therapists, vision specialists, audiologists, and others), special education teachers, durable medical equipment experts, and specialized pharmacy services. CMC account for 1% of the pediatric population yet utilize 1/3 of all healthcare costs, and account for 37% of all pediatric hospitalizations in the US (Kuo et al., 2016). Once hospitalized,

Table 1.1 Examples of children with medical complexity

Examples of CMC	Organ systems	Functional impairments
Trisomy 21	Endocrine, cardiac, and gastrointestinal	Intellectual disability and developmental delays
VACTERL association	Gastrointestinal, cardiac, renal, and orthopedic	Feeding impairments and developmental delays
Spinal muscular atrophy type I	Neurologic, pulmonary, and gastrointestinal	Developmental delays, intellectual impairments, respiratory failure, and feeding difficulty
Cerebral palsy GMFCS V	Pulmonary, neurologic, gastrointestinal, and orthopedic	Mobility impairment and intellectual disability
Spina bifida thoracic level	Pulmonary, neurologic, gastrointestinal, and urologic	Neurogenic bladder and bowel and respiratory failure

GMFCS = Gross Motor Function Classification System, VACTERL = Vertebral defects, anal atresia, cardiac defects, tracheo-esophageal fistula, renal anomalies, and limb abnormalities these patients tend to stay longer and have more inpatient mortality than their same age non-complex peers (Leyenaar et al., 2022). Their clinical and resource needs span the healthcare continuum of services.

CMC are valued members of their families and communities. Despite their high medical complexity, medical fragility, technology dependencies, and functional limitations, parents and families learn to meet their needs and generally describe their children's quality of life as good to excellent (Murphy et al., 2020). Families of CMC commit to supporting and sustaining their children, although that is no easy task. Nearly half (49%) of families of CMC report that their children have at least one unmet need, such as medical equipment, supplies, nursing care, or access to essential healthcare (Kuo et al., 2011). Moreover, 57% of families report financial struggles related to caregiving; 54% have had a family member resign from formal employment to care for their CMC, and 33% report difficulty in accessing nonmedical services such as education and childcare (Kuo et al., 2011). Traditional pediatric healthcare systems that have been designed to care for typical children do not meet the needs of CMC and their families.

Public Health and Children with Medical Complexity

The Centers for Disease Control and Prevention (CDC) Foundation (2019) defines *public health* as the "science of protecting and improving the health of people and their communities....promoting healthy lifestyles, researching disease and injury prevention and responding to infectious diseases." CMC are a small population of children with big medical and social needs. Many public health initiatives have advocated for CYSHCN, driving system changes that have improved the health and well-being of all children. For example, the concept of a patient-centered medical home was introduced as a model to provide quality health care more efficiently. The American Academy of Pediatrics (AAP) endorses the pediatric medical home, which is defined as a system that delivers primary care which is "accessible, continuous, comprehensive, coordinated, compassionate, and culturally effective" (AAP, 2002). While all children benefit from medical homes, CMC in particular need primary care medical homes for routine health maintenance, acute care, and coordination of their complex health care needs. Yet 40% of CMC have not seen their primary care providers (PCPs) in the past year (Berry et al., 2014). PCPs are often limited in their capacity to care for CMC—limited by time constraints, knowledge gaps, constrained resources, and minimal experience with CMC (Kuo et al., 2011; Agrawal et al., 2012). CMC are a small portion of the pediatric population yet impact all of children's healthcare. Considering the needs of CMC when making public health policy is vital to fill gaps and advance the care of CMC and their families in their communities. For example, policies regarding educational and community programs for children need to incorporate ways for a non-verbal child to participate. In addition to merely providing wheelchair access, healthcare settings need to consider altered ways of communication and learning so that all children and families can benefit.

Emergence of Complex Care Programs for Children with Medical Complexity

Community-based primary care medical homes for CMC need strong partnerships with tertiary care systems due to the special health care needs and high hospitalization rates. However, partnerships can be hindered by electronic records interfaces, geographic barriers (families may be in rural, underserved areas), insurance programs, and systems of care in medical and educational settings; communication between these systems is often disjointed, leading to lack of proper follow-up and/ or redundancy of care. To overcome these and other systemic barriers, pediatric complex care programs for CMC are emerging in tertiary care settings. Hospital-based pediatric complex care programs provide comprehensive care that is closely integrated and coordinated with subspecialists in the inpatient and outpatient settings. Complex care pediatricians are uniquely experienced in addressing the needs of CMC and their families, in close collaboration with subspecialists in tertiary care settings. Complex care programs can be outpatient, inpatient, or both, in primary care or consultative models of care. Uniquely tailored to organizational processes and child/family needs, complex care pediatric programs link ambulatory and acute inpatient care in tertiary care settings with community systems (e.g., medical homes, schools) and family services. Dedicated CMC systems of care support medical homes, advocate for CMC and their families, coordinate complex care, and partner with families to define and support care through shared decision-making. Pediatric complex care programs can be high value systems of population health management. They can be an impactful part of the continuum of care and offer opportunities to streamline care for the CMC, limiting unnecessary hospitalizations or emergency room visits.

> **In Our Experience**
> Over a 10-year period, the CMC enrolled in our comprehensive care program demonstrated a 15% decrease in ED visits, 32% decrease in hospitalizations, 68% decrease in hospital lengths of stay, and an overall decrease of 69% in total hospital costs (Murphy et al., 2020).

International Classification of Function and the "F Words"

CMC have functional impairments that affect their participation in typical childhood activities, such as attending school and playing with peers. Using the World Health Organization's (WHO) International Classification of Function, Disability and Health (ICF), a person's impairment is best understood in the context of their ability to participate in their community and desired activities. The ICF model of disability is used to describe the interplay of factors that contribute to an individual's functional level as influenced by their environmental and personal factors (WHO, 2002). The health condition or diagnosis is looked at considering the body's ability to function along with participation in order to complete a desired activity. This concept is taken one step further by Dr. Rosenbaum as he applies these concepts to children with disabilities, which he playfully refers to as the "F-words": function, family, fitness, fun, friends, and future (Rosenbaum & Gorter, 2012). Rather than focusing on a child's limitations, the "F-words" stress individualizing processes that support each child's participation in the activities that are of greatest importance, with goals tailored to individual and family priorities.

Medical assistive devices, durable medical equipment, and skilled individuals that support the function, participation, and engagement of each CMC can enable participation in typical childhood activities. For example, a child with a hearing impairment might use an augmentative and alternative communication device (AAC) to communicate in school and at home, supported by family members who have been trained to facilitate use of the communication device. By integrating fitness, fun, family, and friends into functional activities, CMC can enjoy a shift away from demanding habilitative exercises and toward productive and meaningful activities. For instance, a child with spastic quadriplegia who wants to play baseball might enjoy wheelchair modifications for uneven terrain so that they can join their family or friends in "running" the bases. Creativity and an attitude of inclusivity can overcome many obstacles, while nurturing social skills and enduring friendships. The last "F-word" is future. All children, including CMC, are in the process of "becoming" as they grow and develop. Children deserve a future that is seen positively, without a focus on what "can't" be done (Rosenbaum & Gorter, 2012). Preparing children for adulthood, self-care, and independence is an important part of our care for them. By using the ICF framework and being mindful of the importance of the "F-words," complex care teams can partner with families to meaningfully individualize the care of CMC (Glader et al., 2016). Shared healthcare decisions that align with each CMC's function, family, and environment, while supporting fun, friends, and hope for the future, are essential components of intertwined systems of pediatric complex care and public health systems.

The Right to Education

Like all children, CMC deserve to be educated in systems that are designed to develop their strengths and respond to their individual needs. The Individuals with Disabilities Education Act (IDEA) ensures that children with disabilities have access to appropriate educational services, regardless of medical complexity. Initially enacted by Congress in 1975, IDEA has been updated several times, most recently in 2004. There are six important principles covered in IDEA. There is a promise of free appropriate public education for all children ages 3–22. Every child with a disability is evaluated by a special education team that then works with the child and their parents to develop a unique Individualized Education Program (IEP). The child has the right to learn in the least restrictive environment (LRE), often with special education services that support participation in classes and programs of typically developing classmates (inclusion). If the child's physical limitations are interfering with their ability to participate, then accommodations must be made. The IEP team will explore how to meet each child's needs in the classroom with the goal of maximal participation. The LREs are ranked as follows: (1) typical education with in-class supports; (2) typical education with periodic resource placement; (3) special education with opportunities for mainstreaming; (4) special education school; and (5) special education with residential placement on site. Parents of CMC are essential participants in the IEP development and have the right to approve or refute the final plan (Lipkin et al., 2015).

> **The Six Principles of IDEA are:**
> - Free appropriate public education
> - Appropriate evaluation by a special education team
> - Individualized Education Program (IEP)
> - To be taught in the least restrictive environment
> - Parent and student participation in devising the IEP
> - Procedural safeguards to ensure all students are treated equally

Under IDEA, states are mandated to render Early Intervention (EI) services for infants and toddlers with disabilities (birth to age 3), including family-centered, multidisciplinary, community-based services such as physical therapy, occupational therapy, and speech therapy. EI programs can be delivered in the home or in community centers, based on location and access. Each child participating in EI has an Individualized Family Service Plan (IFSP) that outlines the services, goals, and implementation of their EI program. The IFSP describes the child's current developmental level and measures progress over time. As the child reaches the age of 3 years, the program will outline a transition plan to ensure that the child continues to receive appropriate educational and developmental services.

The Collaborative Improvement and Innovation Network to Advance Care for Children with Medical Complexity

The Maternal and Child Health Bureau (MCHB) funded the Collaborative Improvement and Innovation Network (CoIIN) to Advance Care for Children with Medical Complexity. CoIIN is a quality improvement network that aims to enhance the quality of life for CMC along with the well-being of their families and the cost-effectiveness of their care. The original initiative was composed of interdisciplinary teams in ten different states. These teams included pediatric primary care and specialty clinicians as well as family leaders, public health professionals, and representatives from children's hospitals, payers, and policymakers (Comeau et al., 2024). Key aims of the CMC CoIIN were to increase the number of CMC in patient-centered medical homes, to increase utilization of shared plans of care, to increase family engagement in care, and to decrease the number of families reporting unmet needs (Randolph et al., 2024). A strong national collaboration of experts (Boston University, American Academy of Pediatrics, Association of Maternal and Child Health Programs, Health Management Associates, Family Voices, and Population Improvement Partners) identified a glaring gap in current systems of care. Quality measures were inadequately capturing the lived experiences of families of CMC (Randolph et al., 2024). For example, measures that emphasized function as a quality-of-life measure failed to recognize the valued experiences of each CMC and family. They demonstrated that the quality of life of the *whole* child and their *whole* family cannot be quantified with a standard measure of function. This project highlighted the importance of including people with lived experiences in novel interventions for CMC to broaden the perspectives of policy makers or providers. Partnerships between public health and traditional health care delivery systems are vital to optimal outcomes (Comeau et al., 2024).

Looking Forward

With unprecedented advances in medical care, CMC are not only surviving but are now thriving. It is our responsibility to ensure that CMC have a health care team that is responsive, well-prepared, adequately resourced, and sustainable. As Cass (2020) clearly comments, CMC tend to be "everybody's patient and nobody's responsibility," yet CMC are our shared responsibility. CMC and their families, healthcare providers, payers (private and government funded), healthcare delivery organizations, policy makers, and community agencies are called to contribute to the design and implementation of systems that optimize the experiences and outcomes of CMC and their families. Medical and public health partnerships lead the way.

References

Agrawal, R., Shah, P., Zebracki, K., Sanabria, K., Kohrman, D., & Kohrman, A. F. (2012). Barriers to care for children and youth with special health care needs: Perceptions of Illinois pediatricians. *La Clinica Pediatrica, 51*(1), 39–45. https://doi.org/10.1177/0009922811417288

American Academy of Pediatrics (AAP) Medical Home Initiatives for Children with Special Needs Project Advisory Committee. (2002). The medical home. *Pediatrics, 110*(1), 184–186.

Berry, J. G., Hall, M., & Neff, J. (2014). Children with medical complexity and Medicaid: Spending and cost savings. *Health Affairs, 33*(12), 2199–2206. https://doi.org/10.1377/hlthaff.2014.0828

Cass, H. (2020). The child with medical complexity: Everybody's patient, nobody's responsibility. *Developmental Medicine and Child Neurology, 62*(3), 265. https://doi.org/10.1111/dmcn.14430

CDC Foundation. (2019). *What is public health?* https://www.cdcfoundation.org/what-public-health. Accessed October 1, 2024.

Cohen, E., Kuo, D. Z., Agrawal, R., Berry, J. G., Bhagat, S. K. M., Simon, T. D., & Srivastava, R. (2011). Children with medical complexity: An emerging population for clinical and research initiatives. *Pediatrics, 127*(3), 529–538. https://doi.org/10.1542/peds.2010-0910

Comeau, M., Padian, A. M., Houlihan, B., Coleman, C., Louis, C., Brown, T., & Mann, M. (2024). The collaborative improvement and innovation network for children with medical complexity. *Pediatrics, 153*(Suppl 1), e2023063424B. https://doi.org/10.1542/peds.2023-063424B

Feudtner, C., Feinstein, J. A., Zhong, W., Hall, M., & Dai, D. (2014). Pediatric complex chronic conditions classification version 2: Updated for ICD-10 and complex medical technology dependence and transplantation. *BMC Pediatrics, 14*(199), 1–7. https://doi.org/10.1186/1471-2431-14-199

Glader, L., Plews-Ogan, J., & Agrawal, R. (2016). Children with medical complexity: Creating a framework for care based on the International Classification of Functioning, Disability and Health. *Developmental Medicine and Child Neurology, 58*(11), 1116–1123. https://doi.org/10.1111/dmcn.13201

Individuals With Disabilities Education Act, 2004 (20 USC) § 1400

Kuo, D. K., Cohen, E., Agrawal, R., Berry, J. G., & Casey, P. H. (2011). A national profile of caregiver challenges among more medically complex children with special health care needs. *Archives of Pediatrics & Adolescent Medicine, 165*(11), 1020–1026. https://doi.org/10.1001/archpediatrics.2011.172

Kuo, D. K., Houtrow, A. J., & AAP Council on Children with Disabilities. (2016). Recognition and management of medical complexity. *Pediatrics, 138*(6), e20163021. https://doi.org/10.1542/peds.2016-3021

Leyenaar, J. K., Schaefer, A. P., Freyleue, S. D., Austin, A. M., Simon, T. D., Van Cleave, J., Moen, E. L., O'Malley, A. J., & Goodman, D. C. (2022). Prevalence of children with medical complexity and associations with health care utilization and in-hospital mortality. *JAMA Pediatrics, 176*(6), e220687. https://doi.org/10.1001/jamapediatrics.2022.0687

Lipkin, P. H., Okamoto, J., AAP Council on Children with Disabilities, & AAP Council on School Health. (2015). The Individuals with Disabilities Education Act (IDEA) for children with special educational needs. *Pediatrics, 136*(6), e1650–e1662. https://doi.org/10.1542/peds.2015-3409

McPherson, M., Arango, P., Fox, H., Lauver, C., McManus, M., Newacheck, P. W., Perrin, J. M., Shonkoff, J. P., & Strickland, B. (1998). A new definition of children with special health care needs. *Pediatrics, 102*(1), 137–139. https://doi.org/10.1542/peds.102.1.137

Murphy, N. A., Alvey, J., Valentine, K. J., Mann, K., Wilkes, J., & Clark, E. B. (2020). Children with medical complexity: The 10-year experience of a single center. *Hospital Pediatrics, 10*(8), 702–708. https://doi.org/10.1542/hpeds.2020-0085

Randolph, G., Coleman, C., Allshouse, C., Plant, B., & Kuo, D. Z. (2024). Measuring what matters to children with medical complexity and their families. *Pediatrics, 153*(Suppl 1), e2023063424C. https://doi.org/10.1542/peds.2023-063424C

References

Rosenbaum, P., & Gorter, J. W. (2012). The 'F-words' in childhood disability: I swear this is how we should think! *Child: Care, Health and Development, 38*(4), 457–463. https://doi.org/10.1111/j.1365-2214.2011.01338.x

Simon, T. D., Haaland, W., Hawley, K., Lambka, K., & Mangione-Smith, R. (2018). Development and validation of the Pediatric Medical Complexity Algorithm (PMCA) version 3.0. *Academic Pediatrics, 18*(5), 577–580. https://doi.org/10.1016/j.acap.2018.02.010

World Health Organization (WHO). (2002). *Towards a common language for functioning, disability and health: ICF.* https://www.who.int/publications/m/item/icf-beginner-s-guide-towards-a-common-language-for-functioning-disability-and-health

Chapter 2
The Specialty and Scope of Complex Care Pediatrics

Introduction

Children with medical complexity (CMC) are a well-recognized sub-population of children with special healthcare needs (CSHCN). CMC have been well described in recent years with a robust and growing body of literature. CMC comprise approximately 1% of the total child population in the US, yet account for nearly 30% of all pediatric health care costs, 56% of hospitalized children, 82% of hospital days, and 86% of hospital charges in US children's hospitals (Murphy et al., 2020). The number of CMC in pediatric healthcare systems has increased tremendously over the last century. Since the 1960s, the proportion of children with chronic conditions that interfere with daily activities has increased by over 400% (Cohen et al., 2018).

In 1998, the Maternal and Child Health Bureau (MCHB) coined the term *Children with Special Health Care Needs* and defined the population to support states in identifying and responding to the needs of these children (McPherson et al., 1998). The definition was intentionally broad and inclusive of children with chronic physical, developmental, behavioral, and emotional conditions as well as those who are at risk of these conditions (McPherson et al., 1998). The past two decades of heath care advances have allowed for the emergence of a sub-population of CSHCN. Children with the highest levels of medical complexity and fragility have been identified by various terms, starting in 1989 with medically complex children (Cohen et al., 2011), and more recently, children with complex chronic conditions (CCC), children with complex medical needs, children with complex medical conditions, and children with complex health conditions. "Person first" language was adopted by the community in the early 2000s; now, this cohort of children is known by the term *Children with Medical Complexity* (CMC).

The dramatic rise in the incidence and prevalence of CMC originates from two ongoing phenomena in pediatrics. First, infants born prematurely and/or with various congenital anomalies are enjoying dramatically improved survivorship.

Concomitantly, rapid developments of interventions that address chronic and historically lethal conditions with technologies that support care at home (e.g., home mechanical ventilation) have allowed CMC to live outside of hospitals and participate in their homes and communities (Cohen et al., 2011). The unanticipated consequence of these successes is that we have a growing population of CMC in our pediatric systems of care. The healthcare needs of CMC can exceed the capacity and resources of primary care pediatricians to care for them in community-based medical homes that have been designed for high volumes of typically developing children. In response, a new pediatric subspecialty of complex care or comprehensive care pediatrics has emerged.

Who Are Complex Care Pediatricians?

Pediatric "complexologists" are experts in the care of CMC. The variety of care delivery and payment models (population health, managed care, and fee-for-service) and geographic distribution of resources contributes to tensions around where and by whom CMC should receive well-child, acute, and chronic care for their multifaceted conditions. Pediatric complex care programs are growing in many large tertiary care pediatric medical centers to centralize care with complex care subspecialists and to partner with community-based primary care providers when the complex care programs are consultative rather than primary care services (Pordes et al., 2018; Kuo et al., 2016). In more rural locales, there is higher demand for primary care physicians to serve as traditional pediatric medical homes (Pordes et al., 2018; Kuo et al., 2016). Currently, there is no universally accepted model of care delivery for CMC.

So, who are complex care pediatricians? They may be general pediatricians who work in traditional, community-based general pediatric primary care clinics or in tertiary center based complex care programs. More recently, academic complex care programs are supported by pediatricians with advanced training in the care of CMC across the pediatric healthcare continuum (inpatient, outpatient, and post-acute care). Thus, "complexologists" may represent a multitude of pediatric subspecialties, including critical care (both pediatric and neonatal), neurology, behavioral and developmental pediatrics, palliative care and hospice, physical medicine and rehabilitation, and inpatient/hospital medicine. Competencies of complex care pediatricians are an area of much-needed attention.

Complex Care Education and Training

General and subspecialty training programs have been called to identify the core competencies that characterize a pediatric workforce well-prepared to care for CMC and their families (Kaushik, 2023; Sieplinga et al., 2023; Huth et al., 2022; Murphy

Salem et al., 2022; Kamzan et al., 2020; Bogetz et al., 2015). To date, there is no Accreditation Council for Graduate Medical Education (ACGME) requirement for training in the care of CMC, nor does the general content outline for the American Board of Pediatrics (ABP) Certifying Exam include specific competencies in the care of CMC (ACGME, 2023; ABP, 2024). In the last 5 years, there is increasing attention among general pediatrics residency programs to design, implement, and evaluate competency-based medical education curricula that address the growing population of CMC (Murphy Salem et al., 2022; Huth et al., 2022; Kaushik, 2023).

In addition to changes in general pediatrics resident education, there is a developing CMC subspecialty that is analogous to the emergence of pediatric hospital medicine in the past decade. Innovative subspecialty training tracks are being designed. Over the last 5–10 years, non-ACGME accredited pediatric complex care fellowships have emerged in several academic tertiary pediatric medical centers. Although these programs vary in length, curriculum, and experience, they aim to prepare physicians with general or other subspecialty backgrounds as experts in the care of CMC. These pilot fellowships are relatively new, and their outcomes and impacts are still being evaluated (Cribb Fabersunne et al., 2023).

Emergence of Complex Care Programs: A Potpourri of Models and Services

Medical complexity with multiple co-occurring chronic conditions in a single patient is not a new challenge to healthcare systems, nor is it unique to pediatrics. Adult providers encounter similar issues as they care for growing populations of aging adults with multiple chronic conditions, or MCCs. In 2010, the US Department of Health and Human Services (DHHS) issued *Multiple Chronic Conditions: A Strategic Framework*. This framework included payment for care coordination that reduces avoidable emergency room visits, hospitalizations and rehospitalizations, interventions that maintain/promote function, and palliative care services for persons with MCCs. It supported the development of clinical practice guidelines, best practices, and research initiatives to improve care. It also advocated for innovative health financing strategies such as value-based care and population health management (U.S. DHHS, 2010).

We often see implementation of healthcare innovations in adult patients first and then pediatrics later. Like the DHHS strategic framework for MCCs, CMC too need a framework that supports their care with a formalized strategic approach. The American Academy of Pediatrics (AAP) Council on Children with Disabilities (COCWD) has authored a clinical report, *Recognition and Management of Children with Medical Complexity,* that delineates the need for a system of care for CMC that includes care coordination/management in the context of medical homes, with supports for families and community integration (Kuo et al., 2016).

The Medical Home vs. the Medical Neighborhood

The AAP recognizes the medical home as the standard of care for all children, including CMC (Medical Home Initiatives for Children with Special Needs Project Advisory Committee, 2002). Medical homes have been important for all children and critical for CSHCN since as early as the 1960s (Sia et al., 2004). The current definition of medical home was established in 1992 and reaffirmed by the AAP in general and specifically by the Medical Home Initiatives for Children with Special Health Care Needs Advisory Committee in 2002. In "History of the Medical Home Concept," Sia et al. (2004) affirmed the original 7 components of medical homes (accessible, continuous, comprehensive, family centered, coordinated, compassionate, and culturally effective) and described 37 supporting essential services. In the wake of the Affordable Care Act in 2007, the patient-centered medical home (PCMH) became a cornerstone of medical care, with expanded financial incentives for primary care-based services (Edwards et al., 2014). PCMHs deliver care that is continuous, family centered, coordinated, and accessible. Although CMC benefit from PCMHs, they often need care that is beyond the scope of primary care practices, including hospital services, procedures, and subspecialty consultations. Managed care systems that positioned primary care providers (PCPs) as "gatekeepers who ration care" threatened access (Edwards et al., 2014) and strained family–provider partnerships.

CMC need medical homes, with continuous, comprehensive, family-centered, coordinated, compassionate, and culturally effective care, *and* they need care from larger pediatric healthcare systems. This blended model of primary and subspecialty care is described as "medical neighborhoods" which deliver integrated services in a model of co-management with primary care providers, subspecialists, and community-based services in tertiary care settings (Kuo et al., 2016).

Primary care medical homes with limited time and resources per patient can struggle to meet the needs of CMC. In 2015 and 2016, nearly half of US pediatricians surveyed felt that subspecialists may be better positioned to be medical home providers for CMC (Kuo et al., 2016; Van Cleave et al., 2016), with additional provider expertise, more staff support, longer appointment times, and better reimbursement and support for care coordination in hospital-based complex care programs (Kuo et al., 2016). Although the standards of medical homes and medical neighborhoods remain central to care models for CMC, actual systems of care for CMC vary widely across the country.

Systems/Models of Service

Over the last two decades, complex care programs have been established across North America to address the complex medical, social, and service needs of CMC (Cohen et al., 2010, 2011; Murphy et al., 2020; Berman et al., 2005; Kelly et al.,

2008; Gordon et al., 2007; Cribb Fabersunne et al., 2023). Each program is unique yet typically follows one of the three models: (1) primary care-centered (PCC) models, (2) consultative, or co-management-centered (CC), models, or (3) episode-based (EB) models (Pordes et al., 2018). There are key services common to all three models, including medical co-management, care coordination, and family/caregiver support. The precise details and level of care differ from program to program. In looking further at the general broad categories of models of care of CMC, Pordes et al. (2018) and Morin et al. (2016) elegantly lay out how each model differs in their location, scope of practice, acuity of care, advantages and disadvantages; Table 2.1 is a summary graphical representation of these models of care. A PCC model, for example, can be community based or tertiary care center based, and commonly provides preventative care, anticipatory guidance, and sick care. It has advantages of ease of travel for families, high cultural awareness, and sibling co-visit availability. Disadvantages may include time constraints, lack of skill sets, and insufficient infrastructure for care coordination (Pordes et al., 2018, Morin et al. 2016).

A CC model may be ambulatory based or combined inpatient and ambulatory and may provide consultation for management of rare or multiple diseases, occasional sick visits or emergency department (ED) consultation, dedicated on-call services, or connection to tertiary base services. Advantages include providing familiarity and comfort with complex disease and a specialized "complex-ology" workforce, helping to manage children across multiple hospital care settings. Disadvantages include expense of services, potentially missing children with unmet needs due to enrollment criteria, risk of diffusion of responsibility, and lack of integration with community-based services (Pordes et al., 2018; Morin et al., 2016).

An EB model provides care as a consult team, an inpatient service, or other type of facility and provides teaching or education regarding medical equipment or technology, around the clock bedside care, and acute care medical management. Advantages include the ability to assess and impact treatment or clinic status at sickest time, removing the burden of care provision from the family, focusing on transitions, and utilizing a workforce that is familiar with caring for CMC. Disadvantages include that services are often provided at a distance from family, risk of poor continuity of care between care locations, and inconsistent care teams (Pordes et al., 2018; Morin et al., 2016).

Complex care programs can deliver high-value care for CMC, with reduced emergency room visits and hospitalizations. Mosquera et al. (2014) conducted a randomized clinical trial of high-risk children with chronic illnesses enrolled in an enhanced medical home/comprehensive care program and demonstrated significant cost reductions exceeding $6000 per child-year. Subsequently, they reported that CMC in a complex care consultative service had significantly shorter hospital stays (2.72 vs. 6.01 days per child-year), fewer days in the pediatric intensive care unit (PICU) (0.77 vs. 1.89 days per child-year), and lower health system costs ($24,928 vs. $42,276 per child-year) when compared to usual care (Mosquera et al., 2021).

> **In Our Experience**
> Established in 2010, our Comprehensive Care Program (CCP) at the University of Utah is a collaboration with Intermountain Health Care's Primary Children's Hospital in Salt Lake City. Our model is one of consultative co-management, with an embedded episode-based model that serves with two local post-acute care facilities. Our core service consists of 60-minute outpatient visits, with continuous access to our provider team (7 physicians, 1 advanced practice provider, 1 medical assistant, and 3 nurse coordinators) during usual hours, and to our physician group 24/7. In the last 5 years, we have seen 4000 unique CMC in our outpatient program. Social work, dietary, and child life services are available as needed. We provide inpatient consultations on request. CMC may be seen urgently by our providers or by their local PCPs (co-management). Our physician group has a broad array of expertise (3 complex care generalists, 1 med/peds/palliative care specialist, 1 intensivist, 1 physiatrist, and 1 hospitalist).
>
> Like Mosquera et al., we demonstrated that complex care is a high-value system for CMC over a 10-year experience (Murphy et al., 2020). Specifically, our pre/post analyses showed a 15% reduction in ED encounters, 32% reduction in unplanned hospitalizations, and more than $ten million in avoided costs (Murphy et al., 2020). Table 2.2 shows the empirical results from this analysis. Our position of a complex care program integrated in a tertiary care academic center has been a key driver of these outcomes.

Multidisciplinary Collaborations for Children with Medical Complexity: A Conglomeration of Needs

Shared Decision Making for Children with Medical Complexity

CMC have multiple subspecialists involved in their care. The individual expertise and contributions of each physician and team member brings value, yet it is the collective expertise of the group that supports excellence in care. Shared decision making involves an exchange of information, expertise, value-related priorities, and recommendations among care team members to choose interventions and build common treatment plans (Adams et al., 2017). This deliberate process can improve care and healthcare outcomes in children with multiple chronic conditions (Fiks et al., 2010; Valenzuela et al., 2014). Yet, in a large cross-sectional analysis of the 2009–2010 National Survey of CSHCN, 60% of families of CMC experienced shared decision making, compared to 70% of those with non-complex special healthcare needs (Lin et al., 2018). Measuring the value of shared decision making for CMC is the focus of ongoing investigation.

Table 2.1 Models of care for children with medical complexity

Model type	Primary care centered model	Consultative or co-management model	Episode-based model
Setting	Community based or Tertiary Care Center	Tertiary Care Center	Inpatient Facility
Systematic approach	Medical Home Model	Ambulatory Co-management or Inpatient Consultation	Tertiary Care Center or Other Facility
Key advantages[a]	• Ease of access. • Knowledge of local culture and resources. • Co-visits with siblings. • Preventative care. • Sick visits. • Urgent and continuity needs met. • Comprehensive general care.	• Consolidation of care. • Integration of care across subspecialties. • Connection across setting variations: inpatient–outpatient–emergency department. • Increased resources support—on-call physician, increased care management resources. • Provider familiarity with complex diseases. • Access to multidisciplinary clinics.	• Inpatient service vs. intermittent inpatient consultations. • Focus on transitions and education. • Team familiarity with children with medical complexity. • Opportunity to provide education to other caregivers. • In case of skilled nursing or transitional facilities—prolonged transitions for education, support, rehabilitation or prolonged care stay. • Around the clock acute care.
Key disadvantages[a]	• Obstacles for sharing medical records across different systems. • May have limited access to care management resources and supportive infrastructure.	• May miss children who qualify based on enrollment criteria. • Service delivery may be more expensive. • Services may be some distance from family's home. • Lacking functions for primary care. • Poor reimbursement for indirect care. • Significant start-up costs.	• Risk of continuity gaps. • Inconsistent care teams. • Poorly defined ownership. • Coordination of care separated from clinical care.

Note: Model types are not mutually exclusive, and many centers may have multiple model types in use concurrently. Irrespective of model type *most* CMC models have care coordination to varying degrees

[a] Advantages/Disadvantages examples are not fully inclusive or exclusive for each model, especially when considering blended programs at various sites of service and heterogeneity within each model type

Adapted from "Models of Care for Children with Medical Complexity" by M. J. Morin, J. Alvey, N. Murphy, and L. Glader, 2016, In: Health Care for People with Intellectual and Developmental Disabilities Across the Lifespan, Springer International Publishing; "Models of Care Delivery for Children with Medical Complexity" by E. Pordes, J. Gordon, L. Sanders, and E. Cohen, 2018, *Pediatrics*, 141(3); "Care Models and Discharge Services for Children With Medical Complexity: by Y. Oumarbaeva-Malone, V. Jurgens, M. Rush, M. Bloom, C. Adusei-Baah, M. Hall, N. Shah, P. Bhansali, and K. Parikh, 2024, *Hospital Pediatrics*, 14(2); "The Goldilocks Problem: Healthcare Delivery Models for Children with Medical Complexity" by M. Galligan and A. Hogan, 2021, *Current Problems in Pediatric and Adolescent Health Care*, 51(12)

Table 2.2 Complex care program 6-month pre-post outcomes ($n = 318$)

Outcome	Pre-CCP (6 mo)	CCP (6 mo)	Difference	Change, %
No. ED encounters	224	191	−33	−15
No. observation visits	63	105	42	67
No. admissions	367	248	−119	−32
Total inpatient LOS	3383 d	1077 d	−2305 d	−69
Total hospital cost	$14,708,026	$4,615,838	$10,686,974	−69

Reproduced with permission from Murphy et al., 2020, *Hospital Pediatrics*, 10(8), p. 705, Copyright © 2020 by the AAP

Coordination, communication, and collaboration among multiple subspecialists is a critical part of complex care programs. For hospital/system-based programs, this can occur in the context of shared electronic medical records, formal care/family conferences and informal discussions in shared clinic spaces as well as multidisciplinary clinical collaborations. In other settings, these communications can require more effort and investment among providers, care coordinators, and families (phone calls, messaging, and care notebooks). One model of integrated community co-management with a large complex care program in a tertiary care system demonstrated decreased hospital days and costs, with increased child quality of life (Cohen et al., 2012). The Courageous Parents Network (courageousparentsnetwork.org), an online hub that supports collaboration between families and medical providers with medical information, decision-making guides, care pathways, and share/lived experiences, can support teams and families when making complex decisions in the face of uncertainty. However it is accomplished, the continuous flow of clinical communication supports processes of shared decision making and care coordination.

Children with Dependence on Home Mechanical Ventilation: Tracheostomy/Ventilator Program

CMC with dependence on tracheostomies and home mechanical ventilation (HMV) have the highest levels of medical complexity, medical fragility, technology dependencies, and functional limitations of the CMC population. The American Thoracic Society (ATS) published a pediatric clinical practice guideline to standardized care of chronic HMV, with emphasis on the essential roles of primary care medical homes and pulmonology subspecialists (Sterni et al., 2016). Nationally, 52% of HMV services are part of larger programs for CMC (Sobotka et al., 2019).

In Our Experience
Our tracheostomy/ventilator (trach/vent) program is a multidisciplinary collaboration with comprehensive care, pulmonology, and otolaryngology (ENT) in a tertiary care pediatric center. The number of home mechanical ventilation patients is constantly in flux; however, in 2021, based on ICD 10 data, we were caring for an estimated 223 CMC on home mechanical ventilation, the bulk of whom are seen in our trach/vent program (Kalm et al., 2021). Monthly trach/vent clinics are staffed by complex care, pulmonology, and ENT providers, with respiratory therapy, speech/language pathology, dietary, social work, and care coordination team members that ensure the CMC and families' multifaceted needs are addressed in a single outpatient encounter.

In addition to direct clinical service, our trach/vent program provides continuous indirect support for CMC and their families. In weekly multidisciplinary rounds, clinical teams review the CMC with tracheostomies who are currently admitted to the pediatric care center. The Trach/Vent Task Force, which includes clinical and administrative leaders, convenes monthly to advance quality, safety, and outcomes for CMC with trach/vent dependencies across the system. The Task Force has driven initiatives such as standardized discharge criteria, ICU to floor transitions, hospital to home ventilator transitions, hospital to post-acute care transitions, home durable medical equipment (DME), and provider–family partnerships for CMC across the continuum.

Post-acute Care for CMC with Tracheostomy/Ventilator Dependencies Our comprehensive care program includes care in a pediatric long-term acute care (LTAC) service at a community-based post-acute care facility, which is part of our medical neighborhood. CMC with trach/vent dependencies in need of chronic critical care (stable ICU patients) yet who are not quite ready for discharge home can be admitted to this service. It offers a much-needed alternative to long-term stays in intensive care units. In the LTAC model, families gain confidence in new skills and hands-on caregiving, CMC develop and strengthen after acute critical illness with rehabilitative services, and discharges are systematically coordinated with home nursing, durable medical equipment (DME), and related supports. This novel program has avoided 81% of hospital costs for a cohort of children, amounting to more than $800,000 total per child (Hartling et al., 2019; Brinton et al., 2018).

Complex Surgeries in Children with Medical Complexity

CMC often need complex surgeries to address congenital and acquired conditions, yet each procedure carries its own set of potential risks and benefits. Multidisciplinary collaborations around surgical decision making and pre-operative risk reduction, particularly when considering extensive orthopedic surgeries such as posterior spinal fusions (PSF) and hip reconstructions, are part of many complex care programs. The process is grounded in goal-directed, shared decision making, with a keen focus on the best interests of each child and family.

Neuromuscular scoliosis and hip dysplasia are common in children with severe neurologic impairments such as complex cerebral palsy (CP) or neuromuscular disorders (Allen et al., 2020). Although these children are at high risk for surgical complications, they often have much to gain from such procedures, including improved sitting and positioning, pulmonary function, skin integrity, feeding tolerance and gut motility, comfort, and quality of life (Antolovich et al., 2022). Surgical risk assessments and shared decisions are valuable supports for all stakeholders, as gaps in clinical guidelines and current evidence can leave families and providers making decisions in the face of uncertainty (Antolovich et al., 2022).

CMC are at high risk for complications after PSF for neuromuscular scoliosis and utilize significant cost and hospital resources in the pre- and perioperative periods. In one program of pre-operative evaluation, 100% of the CMC needed one or more assessments/interventions to address respiratory, hematologic, cardiac, and neurologic conditions before proceeding to surgery (Berry et al., 2020). Nationally, hospitalizations for the 5 most common surgical procedures for children with CP (including PSF) accounted for nearly 50,000 hospital days and over $150 M in hospital charges in 1997 (Murphy et al., 2006). Berry et al. (2017b) described the national experience of a population of over 7000 children with complex conditions who had surgeries for scoliosis; they found that the number of chronic conditions was directly associated with median length of stay, hospital costs, and readmission rates in this sample. The impact of programs that pre-operatively aim to mediate risk and improve surgical outcomes are an area of ongoing investigation.

In Our Experience
In our center, a multidisciplinary Complex Orthopedic Surgery Committee meets monthly to discuss CMC who are being considered for major hip and spine surgeries. Participants from orthopedics, complex care, pulmonology, anesthesiology, hospital medicine, pediatric physical medicine and rehabilitation, pediatric intensive care, palliative care, and other services contribute to the discussions. The group considers each child's medical conditions, goals of care, surgical risks, and anticipated benefits, as well as family needs and preferences. Documentation of this process is regularly updated by nurse coordinators. The committee serves to minimize risk, optimize outcomes, and support shared decision making. Assessment of the impact of this is in progress.

The Intersections of Complex Care and Palliative Care

CMC and their families are often navigating complicated, rare, and variable disease processes that do not have clear pathways and expectations to serve as a guide. Additionally, as CMC are more regularly living longer with advances in medical interventions, previously held prognoses may be quickly evolving, placing many CMC and their families and medical teams in uncharted territory regarding planning for the future. With many CMC experiencing changing effects on function and quality of life, as well as potential complications from medical interventions or disease progression, discussions around goals of care and advance care planning are highly relevant to CMC and their families. Pediatric palliative medicine teams are highly trained with special focus on shared decision making with families and other care providers and navigating these challenging spaces with patients and families to ensure that the values, priorities, and quality of life of the individual are held paramount in decisions about care pathways and interventions.

When access to pediatric palliative medicine is available, consultation has been shown to help to increase the completion of discussions around code status and goals of care (Battisti et al., 2020). Involvement of this subspecialty in multidisciplinary care teams is valuable for the shared decision-making process and can bring unique expertise in communication around serious illness, goals of care and preferences in care, and interventions for families and patients at a developmentally appropriate level. In practice environments where this specialty is not easily accessible, providers and patients/families may benefit from the use of several widely available resources. Table 2.3 provides some of these resources, though this is not an inclusive list of all excellent supports that exist.

There is a significant overlap in skillset, education, and approach to patient care in complex care teams and palliative care teams, and at centers where both subspecialties exist providers typically recognize a "spectrum of roles" that span between more complex care based to more palliative based with an overlapping blended shared role (DiDomizio et al., 2024). General palliative care skillsets such as communication skills, navigation of challenging conversations, discussing patient core values and goals, and participating in shared decision making across multidisciplinary teams are widely recognized skills for both complex care physicians and palliative care physicians. More palliative-leaning roles such as symptom management, detailed advance care planning (including filling out code status paperwork), introducing hospice, and helping families anticipate and plan for a child's death are skills that many CMC may feel comfortable with, but many may also prefer to coordinate and collaborate with a palliative care team. Pediatric palliative care and pediatric hospice care competencies were established relatively recently (Klick et al., 2014), and as programs grow, there is increasing access to pediatric palliative care medicine teams and potential for collaboration with complex care teams. Recent

Table 2.3 Palliative care resources for providers and families of CMC

Courageous Parents Network	https://courageousparentsnetwork.org/	Courageous Parents Network was founded by families affected by serious childhood illness and now covers a broad range of topics, focusing on education, community, and advocacy programs to support families and providers.
VitalTalk	https://www.vitaltalk.org/	VitalTalk is a training organization focused on advancing communication skills. There are training courses and resources available for a cost, as well as several free quick reference guides on this website addressing topics such as breaking bad news, discussing prognosis, and responding to emotion.
Serious Illness Conversation Guide	https://www.ariadnelabs.org/resources/downloads/serious-illness-conversation-guide/	This guide, developed by Ariadne Labs with Brigham and Women's Hospital and the Harvard T. H. Chan School of Public Health, serves as an outline to guide conversations about serious illness and patient values. While developed more for an adult patient, it can serve as a valuable starting point in discussions about serious illness for most patients.
Palliative Care Fast Facts	https://www.mypcnow.org/fast-facts/	The Palliative Care Network of Wisconsin has developed Fast Facts, available on their website and an app, with many peer-reviewed, concise, evidence-based summaries on a broad range of palliative care topics. Within the Fast Facts directory, there is a section specifically for pediatrics.
Voicing My Choices	https://store.fivewishes.org/ShopLocal/en/p/VC-MASTER-000/voicing-my-choices	This tool is part of the Five Wishes advance care planning program. It is available for purchase and serves as a planning guide for adolescents and young adults (or adults functioning at that cognitive level) to communicate their values and wishes as they navigate serious illness.

work on these intersecting specialties generally found that practitioners in both fields consider each team's skillsets to be "complementary" and that for shared decision making, often each family and clinical scenario benefited from a patient-specific tailored approach (DiDomizio et al., 2024). Similar to these findings, the experience at our institution is one of close collaboration and communication with recognition of each team's specific areas of expertise.

Coordination of Care and Integration with Community Systems

Definitions and Framework of Care Coordination: The How's and The Why's

A core element of frameworks for adult and pediatric policy for systems and models of service for patients with multiple chronic medical conditions (MCCs) is the contemporary development of care coordination in both localized practices and, where able, integrated across community systems. Care coordination refers to the organization of activities involved in the appropriate delivery of health care services across different providers, facilities, and community resources, particularly through the exchange of information (Kuo et al., 2018; AAP Council on Children with Disabilities [COCWD] & Medical Home Implementation Project Advisory Committee [MHIPAC], 2014). It is defined by four key characteristics: (1) family-centeredness; (2) planned, proactive, and comprehensive focus; (3) promotion of self-care skills and independence; and (4) emphasis on cross-organizational relationships (Antonelli et al., 2009; Kuo et al., 2018). Though closely related, care coordination is distinguished from case management, which focuses more narrowly on managing disease processes and specific medical issues, and care integration, which refers to delivery of health care services that is seamless across the care continuum regardless of departmental or organizational boundaries and is the result of effective care coordination (Kuo et al., 2018; AAP COCWD & MHIPAC, 2014). General principles are reviewed below; however, operational details and execution of care coordination services will differ based on the organization from which it stems. The Patient- and Family-Centered Care Coordination Framework Policy Statement (AAP COCWD & MHIPAC, 2014) offers further additional granular recommendations.

Care coordination for CMC can occur across several clinical settings or community-based care organizations and can utilize various models or tools. Primary care practices, schools, and complex care clinics are examples of common targeted models of care or practices where CMC interactions occur. Kuo et al. (2018) offer several generalities that should be considered when setting up a care coordination system, regardless of the designated practice/care location:

- Care coordination should be team based and acknowledge multiple roles (including the parent/caregiver and patient); however, ideally, there is a designated care coordinator.
- Team should include clinical and non-clinical care members, and staff roles should be well defined and staff efficiency should be maximized with team members working at the top of their license.
- Care coordination should be delivered as part of routine care, whether structured or unstructured, and care coordination should recognize and address psychosocial determinants of health.

- Successful care coordination depends on allocation of resources and support by adequate staffing, training, and assessment tools.
- Practices and systems may choose to train their own internal teams and staff or hire community-based care coordination teams or agencies.
- Tools for care coordination can be utilized, such as process mapping or biopsychosocial patient/family assessment.
- Team members should integrate awareness of the evolving health care marketplace and population health approach.
- Electronic medical records can be helpful to assist with communication and facilitate coordination, and patient portals can be helpful for communication with families/patients (Kuo et al., 2018).

Payment for care coordination and planning historically has not been well financed. Recent changes and movement toward value-based payment and population health payment models as well as greater emphasis on care coordination through legislation and policy statements are better incentivizing and providing increased payment opportunities for care coordination. The DHHS strategic framework for MCCs along with the tenants of the Affordable Care Act (ACA) calls for the provision of payment for care coordination with the goal to reduce unnecessary health care costs, reduce avoidable admissions and re-admissions, and maintain and optimize function. The AAP and COCWD emphasized this framework for CMC in their 2016 clinical report (Kuo et al., 2016). Care coordination is recognized as essential and the standard of care for medical homes and is increasingly embedded in models of reimbursement and health care policy. Care coordination is notably a consistent offering found in each of the three complex care clinic models.

The Benefits of Care Coordination Within Practices and Integration with Community Resources: The Who's and the What's

The goal of well-integrated care coordination is to optimize outcomes for CMC and to provide efficient and effective care across systems. For care coordination to meet this goal, it requires a system that coordinates among inpatient and outpatient medical providers, social and behavioral professionals, the educational system, payers, medical equipment providers, home care agencies, advocacy groups, supportive therapies, and family/caregivers. The medical home is the ideal central point of access to act as the care coordination hub; for CMC this may be a PCP, a complex care clinic, or sometimes a collaboration between both. As noted above, there can be significant heterogeneity in how clinics set up their care coordination structure. Generally, tailoring coordination efforts to the needs of families can optimize support and avoid redundancies. Clear delineation of the scope and role of each team

Coordination of Care and Integration with Community Systems

Table 2.4 Pediatric complex care coordination framework

Clinical care coordination functions	Non-clinical care coordination functions
• Coordinate between subspecialists at the local tertiary medical center. • Assist with coordination of scheduling appointments, procedures, and lab or imaging studies. • Communicate and coordinate prior authorizations with pharmacy. • Communicate and coordinate care plans with PCPs. • Fulfill clinical visits and non-face-to-face interactions both through phone and patient portal in EHR. • Coordinate direct admissions and referrals to the emergency department. • Coordinate with inpatient teams for discharge transitions. • Provide on-call physician paging services after hours, holidays, and weekends.	• Assist with application and renewal of state waiver paperwork. • Communicate with home care and medical equipment agencies. • Provide lists of community resources and refer families appropriately (advocacy agencies, parent groups, charity organizations, etc.) • Assist with adult transition resources (e.g., guardianship resources, application for supplemental security income (SSI)).

member can also be helpful for families as they navigate who to contact for which concerns/needs and avoid duplication of services/orders.

Regardless of who is providing the coordination, key principles of practice include utilizing health information technology and effectively harnessing electronic tools for information sharing and tracking. Use of these tools may include comprehensive health care plans, medical summaries, tracking and monitoring patients via registries in electronic health records (EHRs), and creating actionable care plans (Antonelli et al., 2009; AAP COCWD & MHIPAC, 2014). Day-to-day application of care coordination will often include a wide range of activities including communication with payers and state waiver systems, coordination with local agencies such as the Department for Services for People with Disabilities (DSPD), communication with home care agencies, communication between subspecialty clinics and bundling lab draws to minimize sticks and repeat labs or assisting with grouping appointments by location or day to save travel time for patients, communicating with schools and assisting with school paperwork including Individual Educational Programs (IEPs) and medication administration forms, and documenting and billing for clinical non-face-to-face time occurring through a direct patient portal messaging system or through phone conversations. As an example of these systems, we highlight our Comprehensive Care Program coordination framework as it currently exists in Table 2.4.

> **In Our Experience**
> All patients seen by our complex care clinic are eligible for enrollment in Chronic Care Management (CCM). CCM addresses patient interrelated medical, social, educational, and financial needs to optimize care and is supported by a billing system through the Centers for Medicare and Medicaid Services. Families fill out an assessment tool at each clinical visit which includes their current needs, home care companies, and option to consent for CCM billing. Those that consent have a CCM care plan created in an electronic medical record for tracking of activities and billing.
>
> All patients seen by our clinic have access to CCM services irrespective of their consent for billing; a non-exhaustive list of these services is provided in Table 2.4.

Use of care coordination for CMC has expanded rapidly over the last decade, and as further implementation evolves and expands, we have a critical opportunity to study outcomes and improve systems—especially given the commitment of medical institutions and policy makers to care coordination as an essential service. In the National Survey of Children with Special Health Care Needs from 2005–2006 and 2009–2010, 47% and 43% of parents, respectively, reported receiving care coordination (AAP COCWD & MHIPAC, 2014). This demonstrates the growing consistency of care coordination prevalence in the pediatric special needs patient population generally. Donald Berwick, president and CEO of the Institute for Healthcare Improvement and collaborators, published a widely accepted manuscript in 2008 calling for the improvement of the U.S. healthcare system through "the triple aim" (better care, better health, and better cost). Berwick calls out the critical nature of the primary care provider relationship with patients and the need for a "redesign of primary care services and structures" of which he includes care coordination as a foundational part (Berwick et al., 2008). Healthcare policy as well as coding and billing paradigms has changed to accommodate care coordination in both adults and children. National policy and payment structures are expanding including bigger emphasis on value-based health care delivery systems such as Accountable Care Organizations.

One notable example of a recent randomized controlled trial is a published study conducted by Complex Care for Kids Ontario, which randomized enrollment for 139 patients to standard clinical care vs. enrollment in complex care services involving care coordination. The study measured primary and secondary outcomes that included coordination of care among health care professionals and between health care professionals and family; utility of care planning tools; child outcomes such as quality of life, emotional health, and pain; parent outcomes such as mental health, fatigue, and sleep disturbance; and health system outcomes including service use and health care service costs. The study found statistically significant improvement in outcomes of perceived parent physical health, fatigue, and sleep disturbance as well as in cost outcomes at the 2-year mark, although there were no significant differences observed in a variety of child outcomes or health care system utilization measures between the two groups (Cohen et al., 2023).

While care coordination has become the standard of care for CMC and outcomes of care coordination for children with special health care needs have proliferated in recent years, long-term data-driven outcomes are notably sparse for CMC seen in dedicated complex care programs.

Systems for Transitions to Adulthood for Children with Medical Complexity

Approaches to transition CMC from pediatric to adult healthcare systems are quickly evolving, in response to significant medical and surgical advancements in recent decades (Sandquist et al., 2022). The life expectancies for many chronic conditions of childhood are improving, often by decades, with the benefits of expanded medical technologies and therapies. These developments bring hope and opportunities to families and caregivers for extended time with their loved ones, while also adding challenges and strain to pediatric health care systems that have historically provided extended care to CMC well past the traditional age of transfer in early adulthood. The increased longevity of CMC also challenges families, patients, and caregivers in navigating both clinical and community systems that are generally not well designed to meet the needs of CMC as they enter adulthood. As many as 50–90% of children with congenital or acquired physical disabilities are now reaching adolescence or adulthood, and population data shows that young adults between the ages of 19 and 26.9 years with diagnoses such as acquired brain injury, cerebral palsy, and spina bifida, as well as other complex disabling conditions from childhood, have substantial health care needs and hospital admission rates 9 times that of the general population (Levy et al., 2020). Most individuals report little to no transition preparation before adulthood and generally short timelines between notification of the need to transition and the time of transfer (Sandquist et al., 2022).

There is an urgent need for novel models, systems, resources, and workforce to support the transition of CMC from pediatric health care systems to adult systems. For some specific groups of CMC, there is a growing body of evidence around effective transition interventions. Unfortunately, many of the existing studies do not include or account for individuals with intellectual disability and significant medical complexity (Osako et al., 2023; Sandquist et al., 2022). And while evidence is lacking for exactly which structure results in the most effective, high-quality transitions into adult care, there is clear evidence that structured transition programs have significant benefits for individuals and systems (Sandquist et al., 2022; Gray et al., 2021; Fremion et al., 2022; Vickery et al., 2023; Osako et al., 2023).

The transition process has multiple intersecting and overlapping layers, including medical, social, financial, legal, and educational/vocational. In an ideal system, medical support for transition involves multidisciplinary support from medical providers, social work, nursing, and care management closely aligned with the needs of the individual/family. Frequently however, the availability of transition-focused support varies greatly between departments within the same institution, between institutions, and between county and state structures across the United States. In the absence of a formal transition program, as with so many aspects of caring for CMC, providers should get to know the resources available in their system and leverage what is available to meet the needs of the patient and family as effectively as possible. Creating a transition program can be an accessible and effective intervention within primary care and specialty care environments, using existing models to get started with a basic structure and ongoing quality improvement-type growth as time and resources allow.

Transition programs across various systems of care are demonstrating characteristics that appear to positively influence the transition process including multidisciplinary care, continuity of care, patient-centered communication, transition-specific care coordination, patient/family education, and assessment of readiness (Goselink et al., 2022; Sandquist et al., 2022). Transition programs may also find benefit from including peer-to-peer support.

Most transition programs demonstrate benefit from having a structured process that includes a clear policy and standardized approaches across providers, documentation, and time points for transition stages, though there is also growing evidence to support some flexibility in these timelines being beneficial for some individuals (Green Corkins et al., 2018). Some systems have broad policies in place, and most systems have some variations in different departments. Currently established programs serve as an outline for newer programs or changes to existing structure.

When creating or optimizing a transition program, there are general guidelines that can be followed through resources such as Got Transition® (gottransition.org) and several national disease-specific organizations like the American Epilepsy Society and the Spina Bifida Association. In general, it is recommended that clinics develop a policy as well as methods of tracking and monitoring readiness and progress. The recommendation is that pediatric teams to begin active transition planning for CMC between the ages of 12 and 14, with progressive steps in the preparation process through adolescence and a general goal of transferring to adult teams between ages 18 and 22. For CMC, several key components of transition include decision-making support, topics around funding (insurance changes, waivers, and financial planning tools), educational and vocational needs, identifying adult providers, understanding medical conditions and preparing a medical summary, ensuring continuity in DME and medical supplies, and growing self-management skills.

Decision-making support should center on identifying the least restrictive level of support appropriate for the abilities of the individual. This may range from supported decision making to utilizing a power of attorney to partial or full guardianship. This topic is more relevant in the CMC population and should be introduced early in the transition process; it is discussed in more detail in Chap. 4. Insurance and waivers should also be discussed early in transition preparations, with attention to getting on waiver lists early due to commonly years-long wait lists and preparing for adult disability determination and adult Medicaid applications. There are some financial tools that can allow families to save for their youth with disabilities while maintaining resource limits for federal insurance and support programs, including Achieving a Better Life Experience (ABLE) accounts and special needs trusts. If available, social work can be particularly helpful in assisting families with decision-making supports and topics around funding. The Family to Family Network (f2fn.org) can also be a useful resource, often with online databases of local resources for these topics.

Many CMC can continue with school supports through age 22, with a transition section of their Individualized Education Program (IEP) being discussed and updated from age 14 onward to help with skill building and planning for after school completion. Families may then consider additional schooling, vocational supports, adult day programs, and/or higher care needs during the day at home. Waiver services may become more critical at this age, as parents often need to continue working while their CMC requires support that was previously provided through school services. Some families may explore alternative housing for their young adult through various services that go by different names in different areas. Some options include group homes, host homes or foster homes, semi-independent living arrangements, or more traditional independent living plans. Decisions about living arrangements can be fraught with worry and guilt for some families but may provide CMC with a safe and supportive environment and a graduated level of autonomy while providing caregivers with a more safe and sustainable home life as they themselves age and have different needs. Discussions around these topics should remain very person-centered and focused on the needs of the individual and family in that phase of life. Throughout the process of transition, skill building should be regularly reassessed and supported. While many CMC may not be able to fully manage their care needs independently, many will be able to build skills to manage as much of their needs as possible. This can include areas such as medication management, scheduling or keeping track of appointments, performing self-care (hygiene, medical tech management, skin checks, etc.), and contributing to the household through chores and tasks. These skills can be adapted to the person's abilities and are a normal and important part of growth and development for all adolescents, regardless of chronic illness or medical complexity. Whether or not full independence is the goal, individuals should be supported in learning about their conditions and developing their abilities as much as developmentally possible.

A major portion of transition planning for CMC involves planning for medical provider transfers, information sharing with adult teams, and ensuring continued access to medications and equipment. Families should be encouraged to discuss policies and expectations with each of their providers early on to avoid abrupt transfers or surprises. With some of the differences between pediatric and adult systems of care, transferring to an adult PCP as the first medical team change can be helpful (if needed, some patients may be able to continue long term with an established family medicine or internal medicine-pediatrics provider). The role of the PCP should be discussed, as this provider generally serves as the coordinator or "quarterback" of care in the adult system, whereas there may be a specialist in pediatrics who fills that role for many patients (Gray et al., 2021). The adult PCP can help guide families to specialist teams with whom they have established trusted relationships and avoid redundant referrals for conditions that can be well managed in the adult PCP office, such as hypertension, hypothyroidism, or constipation. With their transition team and/or adult PCP, families can map out a timeline of transfers to adult teams over months or years depending on the complexity of the individual's needs. The pediatric team (PCP or specialist) supporting transition should help prepare a concise medical summary, including age of diagnoses, key surgeries or interventions, latest tests and studies, key trials of medications (and why they may not have worked), and the current plan of care for the coming months or year (timing of laboratory follow-up, medication titrations, upcoming imaging, etc.) (Gray et al., 2021). With access to medical records proving to be a consistent challenge for adult teams, a discussion between referring and accepting teams on the best way to transfer records can be valuable and time saving (Gray et al., 2021; Sandquist et al., 2022). As patients approach transfer to their adult provider, teams should review contingency plans for any unexpected needs that may arise before the patient is established in the adult clinic and review refill availability for the interim. When possible, coordinators can confirm transfer to the adult clinic and ensure needs are being met. Keeping the time between the last pediatric and first adult visit to 3–6 months or less is helpful for successful transfers (Fremion et al., 2022).

Several studies have identified recurring themes that can be addressed in pediatric transition preparation programs. These include building patient/family skills and knowledge around expectations for adult systems of care, understanding the roles of PCP vs. specialist teams, understanding and navigating insurance as a tool to access care needs, and supporting changing relationships as patients transition to new adult teams (Gray et al., 2018, 2021; Sandquist et al., 2022). It is critical for pediatric teams to build relationships with adult counterparts to not only improve continuity and coordination, but also to be able to honestly speak to the benefits of transition for patients and trust in the new adult care teams (Gray et al., 2021). As longstanding trusted care providers, pediatric teams have an incredible influence in the perspectives and expectations of their patients and families. Ambivalence or negative beliefs about adult care and providers can be very harmful to all involved in the process of transition (Gray et al., 2018). It is well worth the time to build relationships across the pediatric–adult divide for the benefit of providers and families with a shared goal of supporting the health and well-being of these patients as they graduate into adulthood.

> **In Our Experience**
> Our institution started formally developing a transition program for CMC with special emphasis on neurodevelopmental disability in 2023 with the interdepartmental hire of a physician trained in Internal Medicine-Pediatrics with fellowships in Adult Developmental Medicine and Hospice and Palliative Medicine. This physician serves as our dedicated provider for most patients in the transition preparation phase. She is part time in the pediatric complex care clinic at the tertiary children's hospital and part time at an adult outpatient palliative medicine clinic where she sees CMC both as a PCP and as an adult complex care consultant. Care coordination support is provided by a staff member of the adult clinic, primarily by one of the palliative nurses with extensive prior experience in pediatrics. The pediatric complex care team remains involved with overlapping requests for refills, DME, and home health orders as patients move their care into the adult world. A culture of transition readiness has developed in the pediatric program, and discussions are initiated, when able, around 12 years old. As patients approach 15–17 years of age, they are frequently transferred to the transition provider for ongoing complex care needs and more detailed transition preparation. New patient panel availability in the adult clinic is limited in terms of both clinical time and physical resources, but particularly in the realm of coordination support, and the hope is for the program to have continued growth. We plan to expand the pediatric transition program to include more formal transition readiness assessments tailored to patients with intellectual and developmental disabilities (IDD), more formalized resources around common topics, and more adult provider options (particularly for primary care). Insurance access is proving to be a challenging aspect of where to direct patients as they prepare to transfer. There are additional multidisciplinary collaborative efforts ongoing, including a separate spina bifida transition program, development of a trach/vent transition program, and a neuromuscular transition program. Several other lines of service, including neurology, genetics, and pulmonology, are referring complex patients for dedicated transition preparation visits with our transition provider.

Transition Gaps, Barriers, and Solutions

As momentum to transition CMC from pediatric to adult health care systems has increased over the last decade, barriers and gaps are being identified. For CMC, particularly those with neurodevelopmental disorders, there is a paucity of well prepared and available adult programs and providers (Sandquist et al., 2022; Gray et al., 2018, 2021). CMC longevity is increasing fasterthan is the development of an appropriate workforce and adult systems of care, causing gaps in knowledge and services for this growing population. As pediatric hospitals, subspecialist teams, and community supports are incurring increasing clinical demands without increasing resources, there is more urgent pressure to transition CMC into the adult healthcare world. Establishing transition programs and connections with adult systems (including two-way exchange of information and resources) can help to address these system issues in access and education by safely transferring patients to adult-serving systems as they enter adulthood instead of lingering in the pediatric world for want of age-appropriate care systems.

There are several programs within the US that are expanding dedicated training in caring for adults with medical complexity from childhood (primarily in family medicine and internal medicine-pediatrics), though far from enough spots to meet the need. Medical training programs are working on including more IDD training, though slowly. The specialties of internal medicine-pediatrics and family medicine are often best suited to care for adults with IDD given the training in both pediatrics and adult care, whether as primary care providers or subspecialists from these initial training pathways. Much of adult medicine is rooted in evidence-based practice with many years of study available to inform best practices and guidelines. Yet the care of adults with medical complexity is lacking in this randomized control trial-type data while the need is rapidly evolving, asking adult providers to care for populations they may not have had much exposure to during training and without well-established guidelines and best practices. Patients, family/caregivers, and care teams are often navigating unknown territory together, which is both exciting and challenging. It can be helpful to acknowledge the uniqueness of this space for both providers and CMC. The average adult provider will not likely be more expert in these conditions than the patient and their caregivers, who have been familiar with the details of their condition for many years. Acknowledging the patient's and caregivers' experience/expertise can be very valuable in the patient–provider partnership and can support development of trust and shared decision making. Providers should be willing to learn about the patient's condition in order to provide the most informed care possible while also acknowledging uncertainty. Likewise, patients and caregivers should advocate for involvement of providers who are highly engaged and willing to partner in this nuanced field of care but also recognize with patience the inherent challenges that providers and CMC are navigating together and remain open to work together to seek solutions. Maintaining connections with pediatric providers who know the patient and their specific condition well can be valuable for all parties, though it is important to have clear boundaries as to who to contact for clinical care questions or medical advice and who is managing prescriptions, medical equipment, and care decisions with the family.

Some of the barriers to successful transition come from innate differences in the pediatric and adult systems in the United States. One major difference is the number of ancillary staff commonly present in pediatric practices, which drops off steeply in the typical adult care setting (Sandquist et al., 2022; Gray et al., 2018). In a more philosophical sense, pediatric care tends to be very family-centered, while adult care is generally very focused on patient autonomy. This does shift somewhat in the care of older adults as family-centeredness again becomes a stronger focus, but this approach is much less common in the care of young adults without medical complexity. This often comes up in communication styles and system restrictions on information sharing without specific forms in place (Gray et al., 2021). Insurance coverage also contributes to transition barriers, with significant differences in coverage of therapies (from a more proactive, developmental approach in pediatrics to a more reactive approach in adult care), access to health systems and providers, and potential changes in home care support and equipment coverage. Insufficient time and inadequate compensation for the type of care needed by adults with medical complexity are often cited as barriers in adult care, as shorter appointments are the norm and care outside of scheduled visits is poorly compensated, along with lower reimbursement rates from Medicaid (Hart et al., 2019). These barriers can make it challenging for adult providers who are supporting larger numbers of adults with complexity to keep practices afloat.

While CMC transition care has clear gaps and barriers, this is an exciting frontier and opportunity for families, patients, advocacy groups, community organizations, medical systems, providers, and policy makers to come together to develop forward thinking solutions. In addition to development of the models, logistics, and structures of the systems themselves, further development of measures to assess transition success is needed. One challenge of evaluating the effectiveness of the evolving transition systems is the heterogeneity of outcomes measured across studies of "transitional care interventions" or TCI. In 2020, a large meta-analysis looked at 52 studies, and patient-related outcomes included impact on patient quality of life, self-advocacy and management skills, transitional readiness, health care resource use, and disability related knowledge (Levy et al., 2020). Meta-analysis revealed some statistically significant improvements after administration of TCIs; however, it was noted that there was considerable opportunity for improved means for impact measurement and methods to increase long-term efficacy of transitional care (Levy et al., 2020).

References

Accreditation Council for Graduate Medical Education (ACGME). (2023). *ACGME Program Requirements for Graduate Medical Education in Pediatrics*. https://www.acgme.org/specialties/pediatrics/program-requirements-and-faqs-and-applications/. Accessed October 14, 2024.

Adams, R. C., Levy, S. E., & Council on Children with Disabilities. (2017). Shared decision-making and children with disabilities: Pathways to consensus. *Pediatrics, 139*(6), e20170956. https://doi.org/10.1542/peds.2017-0956

Allen, J., Brenner, M., Hauer, J., Molloy, E., & McDonald, D. (2020). Severe neurological impairment: A Delphi consensus-based definition. *European Journal of Paediatric Neurology, 29*, 81–86. https://doi.org/10.1016/j.ejpn.2020.09.001

American Academy of Pediatrics (AAP) Council on Children with Disabilities & Medical Home Implementation Project Advisory Committee. (2014). Patient- and family-centered care coordination: A framework for integrating care for children and youth across multiple systems. *Pediatrics, 133*(5), e1451–e1460. https://doi.org/10.1542/peds.2014-0318

American Academy of Pediatrics (AAP) Medical Home Initiatives for Children with Special Needs Project Advisory Committee. (2002). The medical home. *Pediatrics, 110*(1), 184–186.

American Board of Pediatrics (ABP). (2024). *General pediatrics content outline.* https://www.abp.org/content/general-pediatrics-content-outline. Accessed October 14, 2024

Antonelli, R. C., McAllister, J. W., & Popp, J. (2009). *Making care coordination a critical component of the pediatric health system: A multidisciplinary framework* (the commonwealth fund fund report). https://www.commonwealthfund.org/publications/fund-reports/2009/may/making-care-coordination-critical-component-pediatric-health.

Battisti, K. A., Cohen, D. M., Bourgeois, T., Kline, D., Zhao, S., & Iyer, M. S. (2020). A paucity of code status documentation despite increasing complex chronic disease in pediatrics. *Journal of Palliative Medicine, 23*(11), 1452–1459. https://doi.org/10.1089/jpm.2019.0630

Berman, S., Rannie, M., Moore, L., Elias, E., Dryer, L. J., & Jones, M. D., Jr. (2005). Utilization and costs for children who have special health care needs and are enrolled in a hospital-based comprehensive primary care clinic. *Pediatrics, 115*(6), e637–e642. https://doi.org/10.1542/peds.2004-2084

Berry, J. G., Glaspy, T., Eagan, B., Singer, S., Glader, L., Emara, N., Cox, J., Glotzbecker, M., Crofton, C., Ward, E., Leahy, I., Salem, J., Troy, M., O'Neill, M., Johnson, C., & Ferrari, L. (2020). Pediatric complex care and surgery comanagement: Preparation for spinal fusion. *Journal of Child Health Care, 24*(3), 402–410. https://doi.org/10.1177/1367493519864741

Berry, J. G., Glotzbecker, M., Rodean, J., Leahy, I., Cox, J., Singer, S. J., O'Neill, M., Hall, M., & Ferrari, L. (2017a). Perioperative spending on spinal fusion for scoliosis for children with medical complexity. *Pediatrics, 140*(4), e20171233. https://doi.org/10.1542/peds.2017-1233

Berry, J. G., Glotzbecker, M., Rodean, J., Leahy, I., Hall, M., & Ferrari, L. (2017b). Comorbidities and complications of spinal fusion for scoliosis. *Pediatrics, 139*(3), e20162574. https://doi.org/10.1542/peds.2016-2574

Bogetz, J. F., Bogetz, A. L., Gabhart, J. M., Bergman, D. A., Blankenburg, R. L., & Rassbach, C. E. (2015). Continuing education needs of pediatricians across diverse specialties caring for children with medical complexity. *Clinical Pediatrics, 54*(3), 222–227. https://doi.org/10.1177/0009922814564049

Brinton, J., Mann, K., & Murphy, N. A. (2018). *Transitioning intensive care unit patients to an extended care facility: A new model of care?* Abstract presented at: Pediatric Complex Care Association 7th Annual Conference, Crowne Plaza Portland Downtown Convention Center; Oct 24–26; Portland, OR.

Cohen, E., Berry, J. G., Sanders, L., Schor, E. L., & Wise, P. H. (2018). Status complexicus? The emergence of pediatric complex care. *Pediatrics, 141*(Suppl 3), S202–S211. https://doi.org/10.1542/peds.2017-1284E

Cohen, E., Friedman, J. N., Mahant, S., Adams, S., Jovsevska, V., & Rosenbaum, P. (2010). The impact of a complex care clinic in a children's hospital. *Child: Care, Health and Development, 36*(4), 574–582. https://doi.org/10.1111/j.1365-2214.2009.01069.x

Cohen, E., Kuo, D. Z., Agrawal, R., Berry, J. G., Bhagat, S. K., Simon, T. D., & Srivastava, R. (2011). Children with medical complexity: An emerging population for clinical and research initiatives. *Pediatrics, 127*(3), 529–538. https://doi.org/10.1542/peds.2010-0910

Cohen, E., Lacombe-Duncan, A., Spalding, K., MacInnis, J., Nicholas, D., Narayanan, U. G., Gordon, M., Margolis, I., & Friedman, J. N. (2012). Integrated complex care coordination for children with medical complexity: A mixed-methods evaluation of tertiary care-community collaboration. *BMC Health Services Research, 12*, 366. https://doi.org/10.1186/1472-6963-12-366

Cohen, E., Quartarone, S., Orkin, J., Moretti, M. E., Emdin, A., Guttmann, A., Willan, A. R., Major, N., Lim, A., Diaz, S., Osqui, L., Soscia, J., Fu, L., Gandhi, S., Heath, A., & Fayed, N. (2023). Effectiveness of structured care coordination for children with medical complexity: The Complex Care for Kids Ontario (CCKO) randomized clinical trial. *JAMA Pediatrics, 177*(5), 461–471. https://doi.org/10.1001/jamapediatrics.2023.0115

Cribb Fabersunne, C., Takayama, J. I., & Henry, D. (2023). Piloting a new subspecialty: A novel, cross-disciplinary clinical fellowship to care for children with medical complexity. *Academic Pediatrics, 23*(8), 1636–1639. https://doi.org/10.1016/j.acap.2022.12.018

References

DiDomizio, P. G., Johnson, M., & Friedrich, A. (2024). "Who has the relationship?": Caring for a shared population of children with medical complexity. *Journal of Palliative Medicine*. Advance online publication. https://doi.org/10.1089/jpm.2024.0315.

Edwards, S. T., Abrams, M. K., Baron, R. J., Berenson, R. A., Rich, E. C., Rosenthal, G. E., Rosenthal, M. B., & Landon, B. E. (2014). Structuring payment to medical homes after the affordable care act. *Journal of General Internal Medicine, 29*(10), 1410–1413. https://doi.org/10.1007/s11606-014-2848-3

Fiks, A. G., Localio, A. R., Alessandrini, E. A., Asch, D. A., & Guevara, J. P. (2010). Shared decision-making in pediatrics: A national perspective. *Pediatrics, 126*(2), 306–314. https://doi.org/10.1542/peds.2010-0526

Fremion, E., Cowley, R., Berens, J., Staggers, K. A., Kemere, K. J., Kim, J. L., Acosta, E., & Peacock, C. (2022). Improved health care transition for young adults with developmental disabilities referred from designated transition clinics. *Journal of Pediatric Nursing, 67*, 27–33. https://doi.org/10.1016/j.pedn.2022.07.015

Galligan, M. M., & Hogan, A. K. (2021). The Goldilocks problem: Healthcare delivery models for children with medical complexity. *Current Problems in Pediatric and Adolescent Health Care, 51*(12), 101127. https://doi.org/10.1016/j.cppeds.2021.101127

Gordon, J. B., Colby, H. H., Bartelt, T., Jablonski, D., Krauthoefer, M. L., & Havens, P. (2007). A tertiary care-primary care partnership model for medically complex and fragile children and youth with special health care needs. *Archives of Pediatrics & Adolescent Medicine, 161*(10), 937–944. https://doi.org/10.1001/archpedi.161.10.937

Goselink, R. J., Olsson, I., Malmgren, K., & Reilly, C. (2022). Transition to adult care in epilepsy: A systematic review. *Seizure, 101*, 52–59. https://doi.org/10.1016/j.seizure.2022.07.006

Got Transition®. (n.d.). https://www.gottransition.org/

Gray, W., Dorriz, P., Kim, H., Partain, L., Benekos, E., Carpinelli, A., Zupanc, M., Grant, K., & Weiss, M. (2021). Adult provider perspectives on transition and transfer to adult care: A multispecialty, multi-institutional exploration. *Journal of Pediatric Nursing, 59*, 173–180. https://doi.org/10.1016/j.pedn.2021.04.017

Gray, W. N., Schaefer, M. R., Resmini-Rawlinson, A., & Wagoner, S. T. (2018). Barriers to transition from pediatric to adult care: A systematic review. *Journal of Pediatric Psychology, 43*(5), 488–502. https://doi.org/10.1093/jpepsy/jsx142

Green Corkins, K., Miller, M. A., Whitworth, J. R., & McGinnis, C. (2018). Graduation day: Healthcare transition from pediatric to adult. *Nutrition in Clinical Practice, 33*(1), 81–89. https://doi.org/10.1002/ncp.10050

Hart, L. C., Mouw, M. S., Teal, R., & Jonas, D. E. (2019). What care models have generalists implemented to address transition from pediatric to adult care?: A qualitative study. *Journal of General Internal Medicine, 34*(10), 2083–2090. https://doi.org/10.1007/s11606-019-05226-w

Hartling, C., Mann, K., Dean, R., et al. (2019). *Transitioning children from NICU ventilators to home ventilators via a pediatric long term acute care unit: A new pathway*. Poster session presented at: American Academy of Cerebral Palsy and Developmental Medicine 73rd Annual Conference, Anaheim Marriott; Sept 18–21; Anaheim, CA.

Huth, K., Henry, D., Cribb Fabersunne, C., Coleman, C. L., Frank, B., Schumacher, D., & Shah, N. (2022). A multistakeholder approach to the development of entrustable professional activities in complex care. *Academic Pediatrics, 22*(2), 184–189. https://doi.org/10.1016/j.acap.2021.09.014

Kalm, B., Lai, K., & Darro, N. (2021). Care of children with home mechanical ventilation in the healthcare continuum. *Hospital Practice (1995), 49*(Suppl 1), 456–466. https://doi.org/10.1080/21548331.2021.1988608

Kamzan, A., Jun-Ihn, E., & Kulkarni, D. (2020). On the front lines of pediatric complex care: Are we preparing emergency medicine residents? *Hospital Pediatrics, 10*(8), 712–714. https://doi.org/10.1542/hpeds.2020-0141

Kaushik, R. (2023). A comprehensive outpatient pediatric resident complex care curriculum. *MedEdPORTAL: The Journal of Teaching and Learning Resources, 19*, 11319. https://doi.org/10.15766/mep_2374-8265.11319

Kelly, A., Golnik, A., & Cady, R. (2008). A medical home center: Specializing in the care of children with special health care needs of high intensity. *Maternal and Child Health Journal, 12*(5), 633–640. https://doi.org/10.1007/s10995-007-0271-7

Kogan, M. D., Strickland, B. B., & Newacheck, P. W. (2009). Building systems of care: Findings from the National Survey of Children with Special Health Care Needs. *Pediatrics, 124*(Suppl 4), S333–S336. https://doi.org/10.1542/peds.2009-1255B

Kuo, D. Z., Houtrow, A., & Council on Children with Disabilities. (2016). Recognition and management of medical complexity. *Pediatrics, 138*(6), e20163021. https://doi.org/10.1542/peds.2016-3021

Kuo, D. Z., McAllister, J. W., Rossignol, L., Turchi, R. M., & Stille, C. J. (2018). Care coordination for children with medical complexity: Whose care is it, anyway? *Pediatrics, 141*(Suppl 3), S224–S232. https://doi.org/10.1542/peds.2017-1284G

Levy, B. B., Song, J. Z., Luong, D., Perrier, L., Bayley, M. T., Andrew, G., Arbour-Nicitopoulos, K., Chan, B., Curran, C. J., Dimitropoulos, G., Hartman, L., Huang, L., Kastner, M., Kingsnorth, S., McCormick, A., Nelson, M., Nicholas, D., Penner, M., Thompson, L., Toulany, A., et al. (2020). Transitional care interventions for youth with disabilities: A systematic review. *Pediatrics, 146*(5), e20200187. https://doi.org/10.1542/peds.2020-0187

Lin, J. L., Cohen, E., & Sanders, L. M. (2018). Shared decision making among children with medical complexity: Results from a population-based survey. *The Journal of Pediatrics, 192*, 216–222. https://doi.org/10.1016/j.jpeds.2017.09.001

McPherson, M., Arango, P., Fox, H., Lauver, C., McManus, M., Newacheck, P. W., Perrin, J. M., Shonkoff, J. P., & Strickland, B. (1998). A new definition of children with special health care needs. *Pediatrics, 102*(1 Pt 1), 137–140. https://doi.org/10.1542/peds.102.1.137

Morin, M. J., Alvey, J., Murphy, N., & Glader, L. (2016). Models of care for children with medical complexity. In I. L. Rubin, J. Merrick, D. E. Greydanus, & D. R. Patel (Eds.), *Health care for people with intellectual and developmental disabilities across the lifespan* (pp. 195–208). Springer. https://doi.org/10.1007/978-3-319-18096-0_18

Mosquera, R. A., Avritscher, E. B. C., Pedroza, C., Bell, C. S., Samuels, C. L., Harris, T. S., Eapen, J. C., Yadav, A., Poe, M., Parlar-Chun, R. L., Berry, J., & Tyson, J. E. (2021). Hospital consultation from outpatient clinicians for medically complex children: A randomized clinical trial. *JAMA Pediatrics, 175*(1), e205026. https://doi.org/10.1001/jamapediatrics.2020.5026

Mosquera, R. A., Avritscher, E. B., Samuels, C. L., Harris, T. S., Pedroza, C., Evans, P., Navarro, F., Wootton, S. H., Pacheco, S., Clifton, G., Moody, S., Franzini, L., Zupancic, J., & Tyson, J. E. (2014). Effect of an enhanced medical home on serious illness and cost of care among high-risk children with chronic illness: A randomized clinical trial. *JAMA, 312*(24), 2640–2648. https://doi.org/10.1001/jama.2014.16419

Murphy, N. A., Alvey, J., Valentine, K. J., Mann, K., Wilkes, J., & Clark, E. B. (2020). Children with medical complexity: The 10-year experience of a single center. *Hospital Pediatrics, 10*(8), 702–708. https://doi.org/10.1542/hpeds.2020-0085

Murphy, N. A., Hoff, C., Jorgensen, T., Norlin, C., Firth, S., & Young, P. C. (2006). A national perspective of surgery in children with cerebral palsy. *Pediatric Rehabilitation, 9*(3), 293–300. https://doi.org/10.1080/13638490500523283

Murphy Salem, S., Chase, B., Newman, L. R., Cohen, A. P., Cheston, C., & Huth, K. (2022). Perspectives on complex care training in a large academic pediatric training program. *Academic Pediatrics, 22*(5), 867–872. https://doi.org/10.1016/j.acap.2022.03.008

Osako, M., Yamaoka, Y., Takeuchi, C., Mochizuki, Y., & Fujiwara, T. (2023). Health care transition for cerebral palsy with intellectual disabilities: A systematic review. *Revue Neurologique, 179*(6), 585–598. https://doi.org/10.1016/j.neurol.2022.11.013

Oumarbaeva-Malone, Y., Jurgens, V., Rush, M., Bloom, M., Adusei-Baah, C., Hall, M., Shah, N., Bhansali, P., & Parikh, K. (2024). Care models and discharge services for children with medical complexity. *Hospital Pediatrics, 14*(2), 102–107. https://doi.org/10.1542/hpeds.2023-007423

Palliative Care Network of Wisconsin. (n.d.). *Fast facts*. https://www.mypcnow.org/fast-facts/.

References

Pordes, E., Gordon, J., Sanders, L. M., & Cohen, E. (2018). Models of care delivery for children with medical complexity. *Pediatrics, 141*(Suppl 3), S212–S223. https://doi.org/10.1542/peds.2017-1284F

Sandquist, M., Davenport, T., Monaco, J., & Lyon, M. (2022). The transition to adulthood for youth living with rare diseases. *Children, 9*(5), 710. https://doi.org/10.3390/children9050710

Sia, C., Tonniges, T. F., Osterhus, E., & Taba, S. (2004). History of the medical home concept. *Pediatrics, 113*(Suppl 5), 1473–1478.

Sieplinga, K., Kruger, C., & Goodwin, E. (2023). Is it too complex? A survey of pediatric residency program's education approach for the care of children with medical complexity. *BMC Medical Education, 23*(1), 331. https://doi.org/10.1186/s12909-023-04324-y

Sobotka, S. A., Gaur, D. S., Goodman, D. M., Agrawal, R. K., Berry, J. G., & Graham, R. J. (2019). Pediatric patients with home mechanical ventilation: The health services landscape. *Pediatric Pulmonology, 54*(1), 40–46. https://doi.org/10.1002/ppul.24196

Sterni, L. M., Collaco, J. M., Baker, C. D., Carroll, J. L., Sharma, G. D., Brozek, J. L., Finder, J. D., Ackerman, V. L., Arens, R., Boroughs, D. S., Carter, J., Daigle, K. L., Dougherty, J., Gozal, D., Kevill, K., Kravitz, R. M., Kriseman, T., MacLusky, I., Rivera-Spoljaric, K., Tori, A. J., et al. (2016). An official American Thoracic Society clinical practice guideline: Pediatric chronic home invasive ventilation. *American Journal of Respiratory and Critical Care Medicine, 193*(8), e16–e35. https://doi.org/10.1164/rccm.201602-0276st

U.S. Department of Health & Human Services (DHHS). (2010). *Multiple chronic conditions—A strategic framework: Optimum health and quality of life for individuals with multiple chronic conditions*. Washington, DC. https://www.hhs.gov/sites/default/files/ash/initiatives/mcc/mcc_framework.pdf.

Valenzuela, J. M., Smith, L. B., Stafford, J. M., D'Agostino, R. B., Jr., Lawrence, J. M., Yi-Frazier, J. P., Seid, M., & Dolan, L. M. (2014). Shared decision-making among caregivers and health care providers of youth with type 1 diabetes. *Journal of Clinical Psychology in Medical Settings, 21*(3), 234–243. https://doi.org/10.1007/s10880-014-9400-9

Van Cleave, J., Okumura, M. J., Swigonski, N., O'Connor, K. G., Mann, M., & Lail, J. L. (2016). Medical homes for children with special health care needs: Primary care or subspecialty service? *Academic Pediatrics, 16*(4), 366–372. https://doi.org/10.1016/j.acap.2015.10.009

Vickery, S. S., Maturu, S., Khandker, N., Eisner, M., & Twanow, J. E. (2023). Outcomes following a multi-disciplinary pediatric-to-adult transition and transfer clinic at a level four epilepsy center. *Epileptic Disorders, 25*(2), 255–261. https://doi.org/10.1002/epd2.20027

Chapter 3
Community and Family Partnerships

Social Determinants of Health and Children with Medical Complexity

The World Health Organization (n.d.) defines social determinants of health as "the conditions in which people are born, grow, work, live and age, and the wider set of forces and systems shaping the conditions of daily life." These non-medical factors influence health outcomes, and are one of the US Department of Health and Human Services (n.d.) three priority areas for Healthy People 2030, along with health literacy and health equity. In addition to high-quality medical care, children with medical complexity (CMC) and their families need systems of public and community health that support their health, well-being, function, and community participation across the continuum.

The National Survey of Children with Special Health Care Needs 2005–2006 suggested that our healthcare system was not meeting the needs of CMC and their families; 57% of families of CMC reported financial problems, and 54% reported that a family member had to quit work to care for the child (Kuo et al., 2011). An updated National Survey of Children's Health (NSCH) from 2016–2017 identified 1.2 million children with medical complexity, representing 1.6% of the population (Yu et al., 2021b). Only 7.6% of the caregivers of these CMC reported receiving medical care in a well-functioning healthcare system (Yu et al., 2021a). This was significantly less than the 15.7% reported by families of other children with special health care needs. Secondary outcomes such as feeling like partners in care, being part of a medical home, and receiving needed care were significantly lower as well. All these factors were worsened with low-income level but there was no significant difference depending on medical complexity. Even high-income families report challenges with obtaining this care. Both groups report receiving inadequate counseling on transition to adulthood (Yu et al., 2021a).

In Cincinnati, Thomson et al. (2016) surveyed 167 families of CMC for social hardships. Over 80% of those families reported more than one hardship, including 68% with financial and 46% with social hardships. Despite higher socioeconomic status, these rates were higher than families with children with non-complex chronic disorders like asthma (Thomson et al., 2016).

In a retrospective cross-sectional study of the NSCH data, families of CMC reported higher levels of challenges related to social determinants of health, when compared to children with non-complex special healthcare needs (Berry et al., 2020). Poor housing, vandalism, single parent household, poor primary caregiver physical and mental health, living at poverty level, child abuse, parent divorce, parent incarceration, and food insecurity were all more prevalent in the families of CMC (Berry et al., 2020).

Parents of CMC experience unique long-term caregiving responsibilities, often driving purpose and fulfillment yet sometimes pushing families to their limits (Hatzmann et al., 2008). Frequent clinic visits and hospitalizations can strain a family's ability to maintain employment. Some families report limited access to affordable and safe housing with continuous electricity to sustain home medical equipment (Seltzer et al., 2020). Environmental factors, such as rodent infestations, mold, and crime, can threaten child and family well-being. Temporary housing solutions are often inadequate for children with significant medical needs, leaving some families feeling socially isolated and hopeless (Seltzer et al., 2020).

At times, the care needs of CMC may exceed the capacity of their families. Out of home placements, either short or long term, can offer support. It is estimated that about 10% of the 440,000 children in foster care are medically fragile (Seltzer et al., 2019). These medical foster homes can be a promising part of the solution for these complex situations. There are subjective reports that the child's quality of life improves after placement (Seltzer et al., 2019).

Impact on Siblings of Children with Medical Complexity

Non-complex siblings of CMC can experience a wide array of challenges and opportunities. We are just beginning to understand the experience of siblings of CMC in the context of unique and individualized family and community settings. Family structure, culture, resources, and composition are dynamic influences. Siblings of children with chronic illnesses reported more emotional, behavioral, and social problems than their peers with healthy siblings (Quintana Mariñez et al., 2022). Similarly, siblings of children with rare chronic disorders self-report significantly poorer mental health, more strained child–parent relationships, and less social support than their peers. Interestingly, parents in the two groups did not report a difference in child mental health (Haukeland et al., 2021).

Frankel et al. (2022) describe siblings of CMC as a vulnerable pediatric population, observing that siblings were more frequently behind on their well child visits and were less likely to be appropriately identified as children with special healthcare needs than their age matched peers. This is particularly concerning that even within the medical home, siblings are being overlooked and potentially miss out on much needed support and health maintenance.

For many CMC, their health conditions are life threatening. Siblings of children with life-threatening conditions have been shown to have higher rates of health care encounters, diagnoses, and medication prescriptions when compared to families without these conditions suggesting that they may have poorer mental and physical health outcomes (Feudtner et al., 2021). Siblings of children with chronic health conditions have greater depression rating scale scores when compared to children without siblings with chronic health conditions (Martinez et al., 2022).

Families of CMC with tracheostomy and ventilator dependencies were surveyed about their adjustment after returning home after hospitalization. In addition to medical concerns, they report concerns for the effects on siblings, isolation, altered relationships with the community and extended family, financial strain, and need to physically adjust their homes (Henderson et al., 2021). This highlights that these children do not live in isolation but rather in a family, community, and system that needs to meet their needs.

Siblings of CMC often experience *parentification*, with the expectation that they will grow into caregiving roles and assume parent-like duties (Levante et al., 2023). However, their experiences are unique and widely variable, with both positive and negative impacts. Some adult siblings of CMC report lasting impacts on their own mental health (Kirk & Pryjmachuk, 2024) and strained family relationships (Levante et al., 2023). Yet others attribute the experience of growing up with a sibling with disability to their own strengths of empathy, maturity, understanding, patience, and love (Wolff et al., 2023).

Future Directions

Multiple studies have been conducted to improve support provided to siblings of children with chronic health conditions. The studies and the results are heterogeneous, though they show potential for enhancing emotional and behavioral outcomes in siblings (Hartling et al., 2014).

In a systematic review, siblings of persons with neurodevelopmental conditions reported improvement in their own self-esteem, social well-being, emotional and behavioral adjustment, and knowledge of neurodevelopmental conditions through participation in psychosocial interventions and support groups tailored to their needs (Wolff et al., 2023). Again, the results are heterogeneous. These variations may be most effectively utilized when tailored to individual siblings' needs.

In a survey of 91 siblings of children with chronic conditions, 55% indicated that they would like to initiate or increase contact with other siblings in similar situations and specifically address the impact on daily life (Joosten et al., 2019). Specific concerns included worrying about their siblings' futures, handling other people's reactions, and how attention is divided throughout the family (Joosten et al., 2019).

Although there is a growing body of information and resources for families of CMC, research is needed to determine which resources are most effective for specific needs. Algorithms that best match siblings with the most helpful interventions, including games, parental interventions, and peer to support groups, would be novel tools of potential impact.

Medicaid and State Waiver Programs

Children's healthcare falls under state-funded Medicaid programs. In all states, children can qualify for Medicaid if their family is considered low income, but children with medical complexity need Medicaid even if their family is not considered low income. CMC can qualify for Medicaid in two ways—either the state qualifies children based on their complex medical conditions or it qualifies them through a state waiver program. Since Medicaid is administered by individual states, each state differs in how it distributes services to CMC. It can be confusing to families to try and master which state provides which services for each child. When children move and change states, their resources may change significantly, adding additional burden to families. Kids' Waivers (kidswaivers.org) is a resource designed to outline each state's waiver programs, so families can educate themselves depending on their state of residence.

> **In Our Experience**
> In Utah, there are five available waivers for children. The first is the Technology Dependent, Medically Fragile waiver which is for children who are tracheostomy/ventilator or total parenteral nutrition dependent and who have nursing facility level of needs. This waiver qualifies them for home nursing, at-home therapies, and respite care. There is also the Medically Complex Children's waiver which is for children who see at least 3 specialists and have nursing facility level of care. This waiver helps pay for supplies and limited nursing/respite hours. The Community Supports, Limited Supports, and Community Transitions waivers focus on children with intellectual disabilities and autism and provide therapy and community resources for families.

Home Nursing and Families as Caregivers

Advances in medical care and interventions have led to greater survival of children with medical complexity, much of which is due to medical technologies such as gastrostomy tubes, tracheostomy tubes, and home ventilators. While this improved longevity is welcomed by families, there is an increased responsibility to provide continuous complex medical care at home. While most children with high medical complexity and technology dependencies will qualify for private duty home nursing, staffing is becoming increasingly limited, and finding qualified personnel is challenging, leaving the family to carry the burden (Foster et al., 2025). A nationwide shortage in qualified pediatric nurses often leaves families with many days not covered and may lead to significant delays in hospital discharge (Elias et al., 2012). In a retrospective review of delays in discharge of patients with new tracheostomies at Lurie Children's in Chicago, over half of the delays were attributable to lack of home nurse staffing (Sobotka et al., 2019).

Because the Medicaid system is typically the payer for pediatric home nursing care, there is wide variability in coverage depending on the state the child lives in. States where nursing care is approved easily struggle with finding enough qualified staff. This is in part due to lower pay for home nursing shifts compared to hospital shifts. The lack of home nursing coverage sometimes leads to parents having to limit their earning potential to care for their children. A national survey of families of CMC reported 52% of family members reducing work hours to part time, 42% taking a leave of absence, 31% turning down a promotion, 23% losing a work benefit, and 21% stopping working—all to care for their child (Foster et al., 2019).

With this current imbalance of need for home nursing and inadequate nursing available, there is a recent push for creating innovative solutions for this problem. Medicaid funding for children with medical complexity is disproportionately going to hospital care (47%) vs. home health care (2%) (Foster et al., 2019). The hope is to move toward more in-home care so that these children may live at home and interact in their communities. States like Colorado are paying family caregivers to replace certified nursing assistants in the home. This has been perceived as very beneficial to the children and family (Brittan et al., 2023). Some of the state waiver programs will pay family members the respite funds when nursing care cannot be obtained. Since families are preferred caregivers for the child, reimbursing them for some of their child's care may relieve some of the stress families feel trying to care for their child and meet the needs of the whole family. The answer to the home nursing shortage is not simple. Creativity and obtaining input from families will be essential to finding a solution.

Resiliency of Caregivers

When we consider the child with medical complexity and their care team, we must keep in mind the family as well as the medical and social care teams, which include physicians, advanced practice providers, nurses, social workers, and care managers. The resiliency of these teams individually and together must be examined and strengthened as much as possible.

Resiliency is defined as "the capacity to withstand or to recover quickly from difficulties." Caring for children with medical complexity can be challenging, with numerous medication schedules, complex medical equipment, and total reliance of patient on caregivers for mobility, bathing, and feeding. Demands increase when the child is ill, potentially needing additional respiratory support, medication administration, and increased monitoring to try to keep the child out of the hospital. It is important for clinicians to help families build resiliency through positive social support, reassurance, and education. Clinician resilience is also important as they often assist families through many challenging times including end of life.

When parents eagerly find out they are expecting, the birth of a CMC is not typically anticipated (Bamber et al., 2023). Raising a child with chronic health conditions requires that they take on additional duties, which puts them at heightened risk for stress and burnout (Edelstein et al., 2017). Caregivers of CMC experience stressors in all four domains: personal, family, social, and financial (Teicher et al., 2023). Despite these challenges, most parents demonstrate significant resiliency in caring for children with medical complexity (Bogetz et al., 2022). Parental resiliency is of utmost importance, and two of the most critical determinants of resilience are obtaining support from others and maintaining a positive outlook, as shown in Fig. 3.1 (Teicher et al., 2023).

Families of CMC have identified ways that they can be supported in the community. There is direct "hands-on" support, in which others assist with medical care or activities of daily living for their child. This includes respite time, so that the caregiver can perform errands or self-care. Families also stress the importance of "interpersonal" support, where members of the community offer emotional support. "Informational" support can come from medical teams as well as other parents of children with medical complexity. "Material" support includes financial assistance from friends or family, meals provided by the community, and formal governmental or charity funding/donations (Teicher et al., 2023). The ways in which community organizations, medical providers, healthcare systems, and government agencies can support families of CMC are myriad; a few ideas are included in Table 3.1.

Parents of children with medical complexity describe three areas in which they build and maintain a positive outlook (Teicher et al., 2023). "Self-efficacy" is built by feelings of being chosen to fulfill this role or by acquiring expertise through

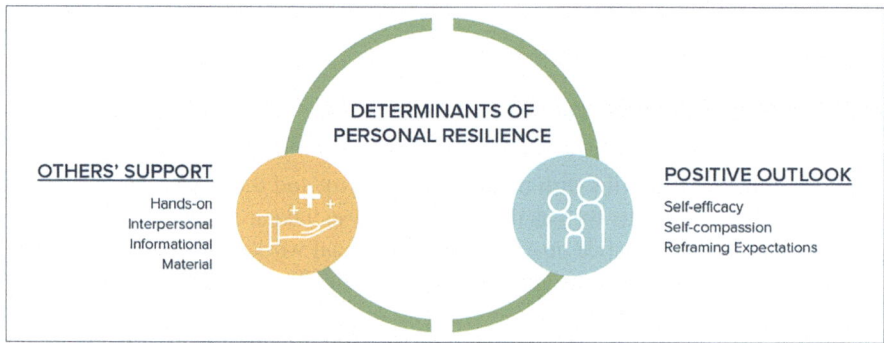

Fig. 3.1 Determinants of personal resilience. Reprinted from Teicher et al. (2023), Figure 2, p. 639. https://doi.org/10.1177/00099228221142102, licensed under the terms of the Creative Commons Attribution 4.0 International License (http://creativecommons.org/licenses/by/4.0/)

Table 3.1 Ways to better support families of children with medical complexity

How providers can better support families of CMC:
• Provide appropriate after-visit summaries clearly outlining and explaining plans (Yu et al., 2020).
• Screen for family functioning and psychological health in families (Scheid & Sahai, 2024).
How healthcare systems can better support families of CMC:
• Provide families with knowledgeable and supportive care coordinators to help advocate for their children.
• Educate clinicians; teach them to not make assumptions and to care.
• Advocate for parental mental health services.
How communities/governments can better support families of CMC:
• Call for policy change targeting housing accessibility and affordability for families of CMC.
• Make accessible transportation an affordable option.
• Pay family caregivers to care for their CMC (Brittan et al., 2023).

caregiving for a child with medical complexity. "Self-compassion" allows them to recognize their limitations and pace themselves to avoid burnout. Families also encourage other caregivers to reach out for support when needed. "Reframing expectations" improves caregiver outlook by changing goals with regard to career, social commitments, and independence which allows them to refocus on the "big picture" (Teicher et al., 2023).

When interviewing caregivers of CMC during hospitalization, one study identified three key coping factors that led to increased resilience: feeling that the caregivers were prioritizing their child's needs over their own, feeling that they could trust in their child's medical team, and feeling that their self-care practices were able to be adjusted to the hospital settings (Krieg et al., 2023). While this was a small study in a hospital setting, the findings start to uncover what is important to families: prioritizing the child, trusting the care team, and integrating self-care.

A great support for families of CMC is the Courageous Parents Network, a parent–provider partnership based out of Boston Children's Hospital. They have many resources available for parents and can also help connect families to support each other through challenging decision-making points in a CMC's journey through life. There are resources for decision making when it comes to enteral feeding tubes, orthopedic surgeries, tracheostomies, and even end of life. A valuable resource on their website is education on how to take care of oneself when your child is diagnosed with a devastating medical condition. Their "Parent's Guide to Self-Care" is an excellent and succinct article which includes many ways to care for oneself including rest, exercise, medication, therapy, and socializing (Frumer-Styron, 2020). In their conclusion, they state, "It is not selfish to take care of yourself. The opposite is true; when you are healthy and strong, you are more resilient and better able to cope with the demands and responsibilities of your life" (Frumer-Styron, 2020).

Organizational Resources for Families of Children with Medical Complexity

There are several organizations, programs, and tools available to families of CMC that aim to provide the various types of support they need. For example, the National Organization for Rare Disorders (NORD) (rarediseases.org) provides information, assistance, and advocacy for patients and families with rare disorders and medical complexity. At the state level, there are smaller groups like the Utah Parent Center (utahparentcenter.org) that provide a wide variety of resources and ideas to families, ranging from local school district representatives to legislative assistance to adaptive hunting experiences and countless other recreational opportunities. In Canada, groups like CanChild (canchild.ca) heavily involve family advocates in their research to help guide the field in applicable directions and to ensure that families are active participants and presenters in changing policies at systemic levels to best serve children with a variety of developmental conditions and their families. Another Canadian initiative, the Navigator Program, was codesigned by hospitals, community organizations, and parents to provide emotional, social, and economic support for parents of CMC (Krantz et al., 2021).

Families of CMC have also started binding together to create change and better support those who find themselves in situations that they have already experienced or are currently experiencing. Parent to Parent USA (p2pusa.org) is a network of parent-led resources and advocates that offer peer-to-peer support, training, technical assistance, and other helpful tools that are found locally. Each state has Parent to Parent programs to help families connect with their local resources. Other well-established groups include Family Voices (familyvoices.org) and the Courageous Parents Network (courageousparentsnetwork.org). Additionally, many families have expressed relief in finding Facebook groups that connect them with other parents across the country, and sometimes across the world, who are raising children with the same struggles and unique healthcare needs.

Partnering with Families

In addition to providing support, some organizations have enlisted families of CMC to collaborate with them in ideas for program redesign and systemic change to better serve CMC and their families. The Family Engagement in Systems Assessment Tool (FESAT) was designed by Family Voices to assist organizations in partnering with families to engage them collaboratively in their work. It opens opportunities for candid discussions to occur between stakeholders about changes that can be made and how to implement those changes. The FESAT was an integral part of the Collaborative Improvement and Innovation Network (CoIIN) to Advance Care for CMC, a quality improvement (QI) initiative funded by the Maternal and Child Health Bureau tasked with improving quality of life for CMC through interdisciplinary teams in various states. To ensure family engagement in the QI work, the CMC CoIIN asked that state teams use the FESAT to involve families in meaningful ways to start creating effective change (Dworetzky et al., 2024).

Many of these resources and tools rely heavily on buy-in from both families and organizations. Despite the efforts made by multiple stakeholders to date, there is still much progress ahead for families, healthcare providers, and communities to collaboratively provide high-quality care for CMC and necessary supports for families.

References

Bamber, M. D., Mahony, H., & Spratling, R. (2023). Mothers of children with special health care needs: Exploring caregiver burden, quality of life, and resiliency. *Journal of Pediatric Health Care, 37*(6), 643–651. https://doi.org/10.1016/j.pedhc.2023.06.003

Berry, J. G., Harris, D., & Coller, R. J. (2020). The interwoven nature of medical and social complexity in US children. *JAMA Pediatrics, 174*(9), 891–893. https://doi.org/10.1001/jamapediatrics.2020.0280

Bogetz, J. F., Trowbridge, A., Jonas, D., Root, M. C., Mullin, J., & Hauer, J. (2022). The impact of caring for children with severe neurological impairment on clinicians. *Clinical Pediatrics, 61*(10), 707–716. https://doi.org/10.1177/00099228221099135

Brittan, M. S., Chavez, C., Blakely, C., Holliman, B. D., & Zuk, J. (2023). Paid family caregiving for children with medical complexity. *Pediatrics, 151*(6), e2022060198. https://doi.org/10.1542/peds.2022-060198

Dworetzky, B., Paladino, M. J., Cruze, E., Fox, D., Roy, S., Bakewell, T., & Coleman, C. (2024). Family engagement in systems change: Use of a new assessment tool in quality improvement. *Pediatrics, 153*(Suppl 1), e2023063424D. https://doi.org/10.1542/peds.2023-063424D

Edelstein, H., Schippke, J., Sheffe, S., & Kingsnorth, S. (2017). Children with medical complexity: A scoping review of interventions to support caregiver stress. *Child: Care, Health and Development, 43*(3), 323–333. https://doi.org/10.1111/cch.12430

Elias, E. R., Murphy, N. A., & AAP Council on Children with Disabilities. (2012). Home care of children and youth with complex health care needs and technology dependencies. *Pediatrics, 129*(5), 996–1005. https://doi.org/10.1542/peds.2012-0606

Feudtner, C., Nye, R. T., Boyden, J. Y., Schwartz, K. E., Korn, E. R., Dewitt, A. G., Waldman, A. T., Schwartz, L. A., Shen, Y. A., Manocchia, M., Xiao, R., Lord, B. T., & Hill, D. L. (2021). Association between children with life-threatening conditions and their parents' and siblings' mental and physical health. *JAMA Network Open, 4*(12), e2137250. https://doi.org/10.1001/jamanetworkopen.2021.37250

Foster, C. C., Agrawal, R. K., & Davis, M. M. (2019). Home health care for children with medical complexity: Workforce gaps, policy, and future directions. *Health Affairs, 38*(6), 987–993. https://doi.org/10.1377/hlthaff.2018.05531

Foster, C., Lin, E., Feinstein, J. A., Seltzer, R., Graham, R. J., Coleman, C., Ward, E., Coller, R. J., Sobotka, S., & Berry, J. G. (2025). Home health care research for children with disability and medical complexity. *Pediatrics, 155*(2), e2024067966. https://doi.org/10.1542/peds.2024-067966

Frankel, H., Matiz, L. A., & Friedman, S. (2022). Siblings of children with medical complexity—A vulnerable population in the medical home. *Journal of Health Care for the Poor and Underserved, 33*(2), 702–713. https://doi.org/10.1353/hpu.2022.0057

Frumer-Styron, N. (2020). *A parent's guide to self-care*. Courageous Parents Network. https://courageousparentsnetwork.org/guides/self-care-a-parents-guide-to-taking-care-of-yourself-as-well-as-your-child. Accessed January 22, 2025.

Hartling, L., Milne, A., Tjosvold, L., Wrightson, D., Gallivan, J., & Newton, A. S. (2014). A systematic review of interventions to support siblings of children with chronic illness or disability. *Journal of Paediatrics and Child Health, 50*(10), E26–E38. https://doi.org/10.1111/j.1440-1754.2010.01771.x

Hatzmann, J., Heymans, H. S., Ferrer-i-Carbonell, A., van Praag, B. M., & Grootenhuis, M. A. (2008). Hidden consequences of success in pediatrics: Parental health-related quality of life—results from the Care Project. *Pediatrics, 122*(5), e1030–e1038. https://doi.org/10.1542/peds.2008-0582

Haukeland, Y. B., Vatne, T. M., Mossige, S., & Fjermestad, K. W. (2021). Psychosocial functioning in siblings of children with rare disorders compared to controls. *The Yale Journal of Biology and Medicine, 94*(4), 537–544.

Henderson, C. M., Raisanen, J. C., Shipman, K. J., Jabre, N. A., Wilfond, B. S., & Boss, R. D. (2021). Life with pediatric home ventilation: Expectations versus experience. *Pediatric Pulmonology, 56*(10), 3366–3373. https://doi.org/10.1002/ppul.25577

Joosten, M. M. H., Maurice-Stam, H., Scholten, L., & Grootenhuis, M. A. (2019). Hearing siblings' voices: Exploring the (online) support needs of siblings of children with a chronic condition. *Journal of Patient-Reported Outcomes, 3*(1), 11. https://doi.org/10.1186/s41687-019-0102-9

Kirk, S., & Pryjmachuk, S. (2024). 'People don't realise how much their past experiences affect them in adulthood': A qualitative study of adult siblings' experiences of growing-up with a sister/brother with a childhood life-limiting condition and their perceived support needs. *Palliative Medicine, 38*(3), 352–363. https://doi.org/10.1177/02692163231225100

Krantz, C., Hynes, M., DesLauriers, A., Kitcher, L. L., MacMillan, T., Paradis, D., & Curry, S. (2021). Helping families thrive: Co-designing a program to support parents of children with medical complexity. *Healthcare Quarterly, 24*(2), 40–46. https://doi.org/10.12927/hcq.2021.26547

Krieg, K. D., Nooraie, R. Y., Favella, M., Iadarola, S., Kuo, D. Z., O'Connor, T. G., Petrenko, C. L. M., & Bayer, N. D. (2023). Coping factors for caregivers of children with medical complexity during hospitalization. *Hospital Pediatrics, 13*(12), e371–e376. https://doi.org/10.1542/hpeds.2023-007207

Kuo, D. K., Cohen, E., Agrawal, R., Berry, J. G., & Casey, P. H. (2011). A national profile of caregiver challenges among more medically complex children with special health care needs. *Archives of Pediatrics & Adolescent Medicine, 165*(11), 1020–1026. https://doi.org/10.1001/archpediatrics.2011.172

Levante, A., Martis, C., Del Prete, C. M., Martino, P., Pascali, F., Primiceri, P., Vergari, M., & Lecciso, F. (2023). Parentification, distress, and relationship with parents as factors shaping the relationship between adult siblings and their brother/sister with disabilities. *Frontiers in Psychiatry, 13*, 1079608. https://doi.org/10.3389/fpsyt.2022.1079608

Martinez, B., Pechlivanoglou, P., Meng, D., Traubici, B., Mahood, Q., Korczak, D., Colasanto, M., Mahant, S., Orkin, J., & Cohen, E. (2022). Clinical health outcomes of siblings of children with chronic conditions: A systematic review and meta-analysis. *The Journal of Pediatrics, 250*, 83–92. https://doi.org/10.1016/j.jpeds.2022.07.002

Quintana Mariñez, M. G., Chakkera, M., Ravi, N., Ramaraju, R., Vats, A., Nair, A. R., Bandhu, A. K., Koirala, D., Pallapothu, M. R., & Khan, S. (2022). The other sibling: A systematic review of the mental health effects on a healthy sibling of a child with a chronic disease. *Cureus, 14*(9), e2904. https://doi.org/10.7759/cureus.29042

Scheid, A., & Sahai, S. (2024). Psychological care of the family of children with medical complexities. *Pediatric Annals, 53*(3), e93–e98. https://doi.org/10.3928/19382359-20240109-03

Seltzer, R. R., Raisanen, J. C., Williams, E. P., Da Silva, T., Donohue, P. K., & Boss, R. D. (2019). Exploring medical foster care as a placement option for children with medical complexity. *Hospital Pediatrics, 9*(9), 697–706. https://doi.org/10.1542/hpeds.2018-0229

References

Seltzer, R. R., Thompson, B. S., & Feudtner, C. (2020). The daunting problem of medical complexity and housing instability. *Pediatrics, 146*(1), e20193284. https://doi.org/10.1542/peds.2019-3284

Sobotka, S. A., Foster, C., Lynch, E., Hird-McCorry, L., & Goodman, D. M. (2019). Attributable delay of discharge for children with long-term mechanical ventilation. *The Journal of Pediatrics, 212*, 166–171. https://doi.org/10.1016/j.jpeds.2019.04.034

Teicher, J., Moore, C., Esser, K., Weiser, N., Arje, D., Cohen, E., & Orkin, J. (2023). The experience of parental caregiving for children with medical complexity. *Clinical Pediatrics, 62*(6), 633–644. https://doi.org/10.1177/00099228221142102

Thomson, J., Shah, S. S., Simmons, J. M., Sauers-Ford, H. S., Brunswick, S., Hall, D., Kahn, R. S., & Beck, A. F. (2016). Financial and social hardships in families of children with medical complexity. *The Journal of Pediatrics, 172*, 187–193. https://doi.org/10.1016/j.jpeds.2016.01.049

U.S. Department of Health and Human Services Office of Disease Prevention and Health Promotion. (n.d.). *Healthy people 2030*. https://odphp.health.gov/healthypeople. Accessed October 5, 2024.

Wolff, B., Magiati, I., Roberts, R., Skoss, R., & Glasson, E. J. (2023). Psychosocial interventions and support groups for siblings of individuals with neurodevelopmental conditions: A mixed methods systematic review of sibling self-reported mental health and wellbeing outcomes. *Clinical Child and Family Psychology Review, 26*(1), 143–189. https://doi.org/10.1007/s10567-022-00413-4

World Health Organization. (n.d.). *Social determinants of health*. https://www.who.int/health-topics/social-determinants-of-health. Accessed October 5, 2024.

Yu, J. A., Henderson, C., Cook, S., & Ray, K. (2020). Family caregivers of children with medical complexity: Health-related quality of life and experiences of care coordination. *Academic Pediatrics, 20*(8), 1116–1123. https://doi.org/10.1016/j.acap.2020.06.014

Yu, J. A., McKernan, G., Hagerman, T., Schenker, Y., & Houtrow, A. (2021a). Most children with medical complexity do not receive care in well-functioning health care systems. *Hospital Pediatrics, 11*(2), 183–191. https://doi.org/10.1542/hpeds.2020-0182

Yu, J. A., McKernan, G., Hagerman, T., Schenker, Y., & Houtrow, A. (2021b). Identifying children with medical complexity from the National Survey of Children's Health combined 2016–17 data set. *Hospital Pediatrics, 11*(2), 192–197. https://doi.org/10.1542/hpeds.2020-0180

Chapter 4
Ethical Considerations in the Care of Children with Medical Complexity

Children with medical complexity (CMC) and their families depend on medical and community systems that are responsive to their individual medical, developmental, functional, and social needs. Yet, systems and models of care vary widely, and connections between medical services and public health systems often lack structure and operational frameworks. Compelling frameworks exist for strengthening health care and public health systems, yet they are lacking for complex systems of chronic disease prevention and management (Baugh Littlejohns & Wilson, 2019). When imagining an integrated medical and public health approach to the care of CMC and their families, models of healthcare delivery (Chap. 2), availability of community resources for children and families (Chap. 3), physician workforce development (Chaps. 2 and 6), and practices, policies, and advocacy (Chap. 5) are integral components. Ethical implications are present in each of these. In this chapter, we discuss some key ethical considerations in the care of CMC and children with disabilities, including the rights of the child, responsibilities of health providers, historical perspectives of the disability rights movement and current issues of ableism, and transitions from pediatric to adult systems of care.

Children with Medical Complexity: Focusing on the Big Picture

The most widely applied definition of CMC includes the domains of complex chronic health conditions, severe functional limitations, substantial service needs, and high health care use (Cohen et al., 2011). Although definitions play an essential part in designing systems of care, they should not be limiting. The process of standardizing a heterogeneous and often changing population of CMC has been described as "fruitful, formidable, or futile, depending on its purpose" (Gerber &

Table 4.1 Principles of medical ethics and their application in decision making

Principle	Definition	Example
Beneficence	Act for the benefit of the patient	Will this surgery improve quality of life?
Nonmaleficence	Do not harm the patient	Will CPR help or prolong a painful dying process?
Autonomy	Right to self-determination	Is continuing to eat with known aspiration the right choice for you?
Justice	Fair, equitable, and appropriate treatment of persons	Of effective options, which medication is most cost effective?

Coller, 2024). The central priorities of care for each CMC and family vary depending on their condition, prognosis, family system, and culture. The "bigger picture" for an individual may involve maximizing function, quality of life, family and community experiences, or future independence, or may involve minimizing trauma for the patient and family and preferences on amount of contact with the medical system. These priorities may shift over time and need to be regularly reassessed. Keeping the International Classification of Function (ICF) (Chap. 1), with its focus on engagement (World Health Organization, 2002), at the center of complex systems of care is a useful approach to keep the "big picture" clear for children, families, providers, and public health systems.

We can best see the "big picture" of caring for CMC and their families by applying the ICF model with a pediatric framework; the "F-words" (function, fitness, family fun, friends, and future), as described in Chap. 1 (Rosenbaum & Gorter, 2012), remind us of individual differences and priorities. The disability paradox, in which able-bodied persons underestimate the quality of life of persons with disabilities, can bias us in designing and delivering care (Albrecht & Devlieger, 1999). We can minimize our biases when applying a framework of medical ethics, ensuring that care is beneficial and without harm, equitable and respectful of individual autonomy (Table 4.1).

Promoting the Child's Best Interests

Ensuring continuous care for CMC and their families across the continuum is a lofty goal in discrete systems of inpatient, outpatient, and community-based care. Unique electronic records and individual communications can fragment care and limit family participation. This may explain, in part, the observation that less than 8% of CMC report receiving care in well-functioning health care systems, in which families feel like partners in their care (Yu et al., 2021).

Most CMC are cared for at home, with families that expertly and continuously address their predictable chronic and unpredictable acute needs. Reliable, high-quality respite services and school systems that include individualized educational and developmental services can support and sustain families in this experience. Medicaid Home and Community-Based Services (commonly referred to as "waivers") exist in all states, although states vary in the specific services offered, such as respite, personal assistance, medical day-care programs, and living arrangements such as medical foster care and host homes. In some states, parents can be paid caregivers for their children. Families may choose out-of-home care for their CMC, including options of skilled nursing, intermediate care, and long-term acute care facilities, residential schools, and group homes. The American Academy of Pediatrics (AAP) Council on Children with Disabilities clinical report on out-of-home care for children with disabilities in 2014 (Friedman et al., 2014) ignited a much-needed national conversation on this issue. As individual and collective personal and professional experiences were considered, it became clear that such decisions are best made in the medical ethics framework, with the child's best interests always at the center of focus. The AAP reaffirmed this clinical report in 2019 and again in 2024.

Decision Making with Complexity and Uncertainty

Many individuals strongly and steadfastly advocate for the well-being of CMC, including family members and medical providers. Not surprisingly, differences in opinion arise when uncertainty, lack of evidence, and multifaceted complexities arise. With the best interests of CMC at the forefront, shared decision making can support all stakeholders. The four principles of medical ethics—beneficence, nonmaleficence, autonomy, and justice—can help care teams and families choose interventions that best align with goals and needs of each child and family (Varkey, 2021). For CMC, parents are frequently making care decisions, given the child's age and functional abilities (though the assent of the child should always be sought when possible). This extends the standards of autonomy and beneficence from the child to the family. Most parents thoughtfully uphold the best interests of their child, in partnership with trusted health care providers.

Effective communication is at the heart of delivering high value care for all patients, and particularly CMC. Conversely, ineffective communication can drive disagreements among providers and families (Rosenbaum et al., 2016). Resources are available to guide conversations when uncertainties and tensions arise, including the Serious Illness Conversation Guide and tools from Vital Talk (see Chap. 2). With a clear understanding of the priorities, values, culture, and perceptions of quality of life of CMC and their families, teams can best guide medical decisions. Some families prefer clear, expert recommendations from their providers, while others seek information that supports more independent decision making. A model of shared decision making is generally preferable to families and providers alike, blending facts, opinions, and emotions to reach clear decisions and plans (Racine, 2016).

Patients, families, and providers carry personal religious, cultural, professional, and historical experiences to each situation, which influence recommendations in the decisions being made. Providers may bring their own personal preferences and professional experiences to specific cases/situations. Similarly, families bring their own experiences, beliefs, values, and hopes into complex decision-making processes. CMC too may have values and preferences about a decision, even when limited by decision-making capacity and authority. The input of each team member should be considered as teams make decisions in the child's best interest, incorporating a shared understanding of the benefits and burdens of available options in the context of the values and goals of each child and family. Providers have a responsibility to be aware of personal biases which may affect discussions with families and keep an objective approach to care. Families and providers can find decision support though care conferences, confidential consultations with colleagues, conversations with trusted stakeholders, and consultations with multidisciplinary ethics committees as needed. The American Academy of Pediatrics recommends that ethics committees within institutions be an available, accessible resource to patients, families, providers, and staff when addressing ethical dilemmas and challenging decisions (Moon et al., 2019). If a provider is unable to follow a joint plan in good conscience, they should recuse themselves from further involvement. If a joint plan cannot be tolerated by any party, the case may require transfer to another institution (if a receiving institution can be identified, which is rare) or the judicial system may need to become involved (Needelman & Sweeney, 2016).

What Is the Right "Dose" of Care?

Overutilization, overdiagnosis, overtreatment—these and similar terms are important when considering the care of CMC. Pediatricians for CMC often find themselves making treatment decisions without clear evidence and clinical guidelines. Well-intended providers and parents may feel compelled to do something, as the alternative can be uncomfortable. This all-too-familiar scenario can lead to overmedicalization, driven by parental worry and provider distress (Rosenbaum et al., 2016). In extreme instances, medical child abuse can occur.

Medical child abuse (previously known as Munchausen by proxy) is a form of child maltreatment in which a child is subjected to unnecessary and harmful or potentially harmful care at the request of the parent/caregiver. Over-medicalization by worried parents becomes medical child abuse when there is real or potential harm to the child. Discrépancies between histories and direct observations, the provision of a large amount of healthcare without desired outcomes, and parent-directed consultations with multiple providers and subspecialists can alert providers to the possibility that over-medicalization is approaching medical child abuse.

Families may opt to care for their CMC by primarily addressing symptoms and declining invasive or potentially uncomfortable hospital admissions and related interventions. Providers may be tempted to interpret this as non-compliance and intentional disregard for medical recommendations, while parents may be balancing goals for their child and family in the context of their culture, values, and resources (Phoenix, 2016). Parent and provider goals can differ without concerns for neglect. When intervention is futile, as with any other decisions in care, parents can make decisions that align with their values, goals, and priorities while providers also uphold their own values without compromise of principles. Consultations with colleagues, ethics committees, and palliative care teams can support providers and parents in developing personal resuscitation plans for CMC (Newman & Zurbrugg, 2016). At times, questions of acceptable family care choices can stretch the abilities of even the most capable, educated, and well-intentioned medical professionals, and can raise questions of abuse and neglect. As mandatory reporters, providers must protect vulnerable members of society and maintain the best interests of each child. Although providers may feel conflicted reporting to child protection services (CPS), these agencies can broadly assess concerns for medical abuse and neglect and also connect families with additional community and social supports for the CMC and entire family (Lach & Birnbaum, 2016).

Again, principles of medical ethics and shared decision making can support providers and families when facing uncertainty regarding the care of CMC. The best interests of the child, with an understanding of quality of life and comfort in the context of family values, personal definitions of quality of life, and culture, can keep the focus clear. The spectrum of acceptable parental decision making is broad, and parent–provider partnerships can limit over- and under-medicalization, and at the extremes, medical abuse and neglect.

Growth Attenuation Therapy: An Example of Shared Decision Making

When CMC have permanent and profound physical and cognitive disabilities, the physical demands of caregiving tend to increase as children approach adult size and their parents age. For some families, out-of-home placements are necessary. For others, strategies that limit physical growth can sustain family caregiving for CMC in their homes and communities. Growth attenuation therapy (GAT) can limit the physical growth of children with profound physical and cognitive disabilities. High doses of estrogen accelerate the closure of growth plates and reduce the child's final adult height. This can proceed endogenously, by allowing precocious puberty to advance naturally, or by administering exogenous estrogen.

This treatment captured national attention with the case of Ashley X, a child with severe disabilities whose parents opted for GAT to sustain caring for her at home, raising many aspects of the care of CMC to broader attention and discussion (Gunther & Diekema, 2006; Coombes, 2007). As this case illustrated, this approach demands consideration in a bioethical framework, as it has potential implications for child autonomy, quality of life, long-term health effects, and societal implications (altering the individual to fit societal norms). From a purely scientific approach, GAT is a safe and beneficial option for certain families. With a medically reasonable choice such as GAT, the ethical considerations for a family become the most important determinant in a choice to utilize or decline this treatment. Depending on the perspectives of any given family, this treatment may be fully aligned with goals of allowing their CMC to be cared for more easily in the home or could run contrary to their priority of preserving their child's physical autonomy. This is where shared decision-making approaches can support parents and providers in exploring the risks and benefits of GAT for their child and family. Parents and providers generally agree that treatment decisions should promote the best interests of each CMC; yet they also need to agree on how to best achieve this goal. Without any single standard algorithm or one-size-fits-all guideline, shared decision making with all stakeholders remains the best approach to difficult, sensitive, personal, and complex healthcare decisions for CMC.

Complementary and Alternative Medicine

As famously stated, the "absence of evidence is not evidence of absence." Complementary and alternative medicine (CAM) continues to evolve with growing evidence for or against the efficacy of various interventions as those with supporting evidence becoming more integrated into mainstream western medicine. Particularly in areas without clear paths to cure and without robust evidence-based guidelines and treatments, families may seek out additional treatment options and wish to incorporate CAM into their child's plan of care (Hurvitz & Noritz, 2016; Akins et al., 2014). Providers can talk with families to understand the basis for these requests and assess the risks and benefits objectively before making treatment recommendations. The spoken and unspoken motivations for seeking CAM may include frustration with a lack of available treatments and research, known risks with standard treatments, social and cultural backgrounds, and the sincere desire to help children heal, grow, and feel well (Hurvitz & Noritz, 2016; Grossberg, 2008). With open minded, non-judgmental communications, providers and families can align their goals of supporting the child's best interests when making CAM treatment decisions.

A blanket "yes" or "no" approach to alternative therapies (including supplements, herbal remedies, aromatherapy, essential oils, etc.) will likely leave out important considerations around safety as well as potential benefit. Known risks, such as medication interactions and bleeding risk with supplements or toxicity with essential oils, as well as individual risks, such as orthopedic contraindications to chiropractic manipulation or seizure risk with cannabis, should be considered. The financial and resource implications should also be taken into account. Providers should not feel pressured to write letters of support or prescriptions for treatments they do not feel are in the best interest of the child (Bell et al., 2011). However, if the balance between risk and benefit is favorable or even neutral, it may be worth supporting a trial of an intervention with careful observation by families and providers. Together, they can assess outcomes and decide on duration of interventions (Hurvitz & Noritz, 2016). This may not only benefit the patient with desired effects but also build trust with families as an active part of the child's team and facilitate ongoing honest discussions of future treatment plans, both traditional and nontraditional, within western medicine practice. Providers should remain open to discussions and new evidence as they care for CMC.

Decision Making, Autonomy, and Support in the Transition to Adulthood

As CMC approach adulthood, changes in legal status, decision-making supports, and confidentiality become important elements of care. In most states, individuals are considered adults at age 18, with the rights and responsibilities associated with that legal status. For CMC, there may be experiential and developmental reasons that they are not ready or able to function independently when they reach 18 years (Sufian et al., 2018). Many young adults may be able to learn and develop skills to take on more independence over time, requiring some support that may eventually wane. Others may have intellectual and developmental disabilities that permanently affect their ability to independently manage their care needs. Caregivers and providers should support individuals in developing their independence to the best of their abilities, even if that does not mean full self-management, and utilize the least restrictive support options to protect the safety and well-being of adults with medical complexity and developmental disabilities (Turchi et al., 2024).

There are multiple tools available to support adults who need assistance with decision making, ranging from information release forms to full legal guardianship. Some of these tools come into play when the individual temporarily loses capacity to make certain decisions, while others are permanently in place based on a determination of competency. Capacity refers to a person's ability to perform a specific task and can vary depending on the type of task and on modifiable conditions. For example, an individual may have capacity to participate in some decisions like the day/time of appointments but not in more complex decisions like surgical consents or end-of-life plans. They may have the capacity to make decisions most of the time but lack capacity when they are encephalopathic after seizures or when acutely ill. To demonstrate capacity, the individual must be able to understand the situation and relevant information, reason through risks and benefits of options, and express a consistent choice. Capacity does not mean that the person agrees with their provider or caregiver but that they can make a rational choice based on their own thought processes and values (Chuang & Kennedy, 2016; Turchi et al., 2024). Competence refers to a legal determination of a person's ability to make decisions and is not routinely subject to changes without additional legal action (Sufian et al., 2018). Neuropsychological testing, Individual Education Program (IEP) reports, and input from caregivers, therapists, teachers, and medical providers can help to determine the strengths and deficits in a person's cognitive abilities, thus guiding what level of support is appropriate.

Guardianship is a legal process that fully substitutes an individual's decision-making authority, placing that responsibility with the person's guardian. This is the most restrictive form of decision-making support and should be reserved for individuals who do not have the ability to safely manage their own medical, financial, and personal decisions and care. It functions similarly to parental rights of minors, with permission required from the guardian for medical interventions and legal agreements such as leases and contracts. Areas affected by guardianship can include medical decisions, finances, living arrangements, ability to possess a driver's license, marry, vote, or possess a firearm (Chuang & Kennedy, 2016). Guardianship is called conservatorship in some states, and there can be partial or full guardianship depending on which aspects of a person's life require substituted decision making. The process of applying for guardianship varies significantly between states and may or may not require medical assessments, psychological testing, and involvement of an attorney (Chuang & Kennedy, 2016; Turchi et al., 2024). Cost can also vary significantly and may pose a significant barrier to some families. Even with fully substituted medical decision making through guardianship, the individual should be involved in their care and decisions as much as possible, and their preferences should be respected whenever safe and reasonable, maximizing their functional autonomy even when legal autonomy cannot be safely preserved.

Supported Decision Making (SDM) is a tool that can aid individuals needing assistance with decisions in certain instances but who are generally capable of managing their own decisions and needs. This tool is legally in place in some states and becoming more available in others. SDM involves the individual identifying areas where they would like support, who they want to help them, and how they want that help (Chuang & Kennedy, 2016; Sufian et al., 2018). This information is documented in a SDM agreement that can then be shared with medical teams to use when appropriate. An example would be a young adult requesting support from the mother and older sister when they have medical appointments and procedures. They may ask the team to prepare a detailed visit summary to share with their supporters or have these people present for visits and consent discussions (Turchi et al., 2024). The supporters can help to make sure the individual is considering the right information and goals as they come to their decision. In SDM, the decisions rest with the individual, who uses their support system for specific needs. As the individual grows in experience and confidence, they may be able to reduce the support they need.

There are several other tools in the continuum of decision-making supports that go by various terms in different systems and states. Young adults can sign releases to allow trusted adults (parents or otherwise) to access their medical information and help with scheduling appointments, etc. They can also assign a power of attorney or healthcare proxy, which allows a designated adult to make decisions for the individual in specific circumstances, often in the event of losing capacity. The individual must have capacity to make this decision when the required form is completed (Sufian et al., 2018). This may be included in some advance care planning documentation. Individuals may choose to utilize joint bank accounts or a living trust for financial and property management support (Chuang & Kennedy, 2016; Turchi et al., 2024).

Confidentiality and consent are additional important aspects of the care of adolescents and young adults, with some nuances for individuals with intellectual and developmental disabilities (IDD). Providers should become familiar with the laws around confidentiality and consent for minors in their state and healthcare system, as these can vary significantly. For many adolescents, these concepts become particularly relevant around topics including reproductive health, substance use and misuse, sexual identity and gender orientation, and risk-taking behaviors. These topics are relevant for youth with IDD as much as their neurotypical peers, though often not addressed as consistently by providers. For young adults who have guardianship in place, privacy should still be considered and respected whenever possible. Adolescents as well as adults with guardianship in place may not be able to provide informed consent, but they can and should be encouraged to participate in discussions and share their assent or dissent to participate in plans of care whenever possible. Through the lens of ethics, individuals with IDD and medical complexity should have their autonomy, privacy, and values understood and supported as consistently as possible to the extent possible in the context of their medical, cognitive, and social needs and abilities.

In Our Experience
We launched a structured healthcare transition program for CMC in 2023. We introduce transitions by age 16 and support patients in transferring to adult providers between 18 and 21 years of age. We find that many families are anxious about the prospect of transition but have not had outlets to discuss and prepare. Most families benefit from a stepwise approach, starting with completion of waiver applications, and then preparing for decision-making supports, adult insurance changes and Supplemental Security Income (SSI), and detailed plans for medical transitions. The needs of families vary widely. For patients on the borderline of needing guardianship versus a less restrictive option, seeking our neuropsychological testing can be helpful to delineate cognitive strengths and deficits. Efforts to find welcoming adult providers have been well worth the time, establishing reliable referral networks to put both providers and families at ease through a process of change that can naturally bring uncertainty.

Table 4.2 provides additional information and resources that may be helpful for providers as well as families about transitions for individuals with IDD and medical complexity, including decision-making support, readiness assessments, and topics to address in the transition phase.

Advance care planning can be integrated into discussions about transition to adult systems of care. For many CMC, these topics have been addressed periodically throughout childhood. Providers can utilize palliative medicine teams when available to aid in these discussions. The overarching goals of care or priorities in care should be reviewed often, deciding on each individual's ideal balance of

Table 4.2 Decision-making support and transition to adult care resources

National Resource Center for Supported Decision Making	https://supporteddecisionmaking.org/
Utah Parent Center Family to Family Network	https://utahparentcenter.org/guardianship/
Vanderbilt IDD Toolkit	https://iddtoolkit.vkcsites.org/
American College of Physicians Pediatric to Adult Care Transitions Initiative	https://www.acponline.org/clinical-information/high-value-care/resources-for-clinicians/pediatric-to-adult-care-transitions-initiative
Got Transition® for Special Populations	https://www.gottransition.org/resources-and-research/special-populations.cfm
Spina Bifida Association Transition Guideline	https://www.spinabifidaassociation.org/resource/transition/
American Epilepsy Society Clinical Practice Tools	https://aesnet.org/clinical-care/running-your-practice
Center for Transition to Adult Health Care for Youth with Disabilities	https://movingtoadulthealthcare.org/toolkits/

quality and quantity of life. Interventions can then be evaluated in the context of what is most important to each person. Individuals and families may not have any limits on future interventions or may have certain things that are not acceptable, such as cardiopulmonary resuscitation, intubation, artificial nutrition, complex surgeries, or even future hospital admissions. These preferences may change over time and should be routinely reviewed to understand and support changes. For those who identify limits to future interventions, a Physician Orders for Life-Sustaining Treatment (POLST) form or the equivalent (e.g., Physician Orders for Scope of Treatment, Medical Orders for Life-Sustaining Treatment) may be useful in community settings. In addition to reviewing quality of life and whether any limits on future interventions are appropriate, advance care planning should include considerations of who will support the young adult in the event of their caregivers no longer being able to support them due to injury, illness, or death. This often involves addressing with families a will or trust, guardianship succession planning, and financial planning (this may include ABLE accounts or a Special Needs Trust, tools specifically designed for adults with IDD and complexity). Discussions around transition can be a nice opening to ensure that families are considering these future plans and hopefully allow for discussions well before they are urgent or emergent in nature.

For some adolescents and young adults with medical complexity and life-limiting conditions, transition to adult care may not be the right decision. While it is appropriate to standardize transition policies for most CMC, providers should allow flexibility on timelines for those who are near their end of life. The process of transferring to new care teams and institutions can be stressful and challenging in the best of scenarios, and pushing these changes in times of serious illness or crisis can augment trauma for patients, families, and even providers and worsen gaps in care. Extending pediatric services may also be appropriate for some rare conditions that can only be safely managed by a small group of pediatric providers or for individuals with very small stature, as weight-based dosing is much less commonly utilized in adult care and may pose a safety concern without adequate preparation in the new adult system. Families should be involved in conversations about all aspects of transition, including when it may be appropriate to postpone or forego transfers.

Children with Medical Complexity: US Disability Rights and Challenges

The disability rights movement in the United States (US) has spanned over 200 years, and yet there still is more to be done. In 1815, educational programs for deaf students were implemented, followed closely by the invention of the Braille alphabet in 1829. Yet, not until Franklin D. Roosevelt (FDR), paralyzed by polio, was elected president (1932) did we see widespread support for persons with disabilities. FDR signed the Social Security Act in 1935, ensuring assistance for adults with disabilities in the US. After World War II, the Veterans Administration (VA) ignited advocacy for barrier-free communities and the civil rights of veterans with disabilities. In the 1950s, school segregation was abolished, and children with intellectual disabilities were educated in public school systems. The Civil Rights Act of 1964 was passed to prevent discrimination based on race, sex, national origin, age, and religion, yet it did not make any provision for people with disabilities.

The first major US legislation supporting the rights of persons with disabilities was the Rehabilitation Act of 1973, including Section 504. This historic shift in public policy for people with disabilities prohibits discrimination based on disability in federally supported programs. It guarantees equal opportunity in federally funded programs, including employment, public housing, transportation, and vocational training programs. This was quickly followed by the Education for All Handicapped Children Act in 1975, guaranteeing equal access to free, appropriate public education (FAPE) for children with disabilities in the least restrictive environment. In 1990, this act was renamed the Individuals with Disabilities Education Act (IDEA), with the addition of the inclusive participation of parents in making educational decisions for their children with disabilities, including the development of Individual Education Programs (IEPs).

Decades of individual and collective civil rights advocacy culminated in the signing of the Americans with Disabilities Act (ADA) in 1990. President George H.W. Bush signed the act into law, stating, "Let the shameful wall of exclusion finally come tumbling down" (Bush, 2016). The ADA prohibits disability discrimination in employment, services rendered by state and local governments, and places of public accommodation, transportation, and telecommunications services. It requires reasonable accommodations and modifications that support inclusion and participation of people with disabilities. The ADA was amended in 2008 to broaden the definition of disability and protect individuals with impairments related to chronic conditions such as cancer, diabetes, and epilepsy. These legislative milestones have significantly expanded the legal protections for people with disabilities. At the same time, ableism—discrimination in favor of able-bodied people—exists and warrants further action.

Internationally, the United Nations (UN) Declaration of the Rights of the Child in 1959 stated that all children have rights to protection, education, health care, shelter, and good nutrition. At the 20th anniversary of this declaration (1979), the Convention of the Rights of the Child was published and then adopted by the United Nations General Assembly in 1989. This document defines universal rights for all children, including protection from discrimination, prioritizing the best interests of the child, protecting the safety, health, development, and identity of children, keeping families together when safe and possible to do so, and protecting freedoms around thoughts, religion, culture, opinions, and choices. Specifically, children with disabilities have the right to enjoy the best possible life in society, with active community participation. The Convention of the Rights of the Child is the most widely ratified human rights treaty in the world. In 2009, President Barack Obama signed the UN Convention on the Rights of People with Disabilities to promote and protect the equal enjoyment of human rights and dignity of all people.

Ableism: A Modern-Day Issue for Children with Medical Complexity

The historical backdrop of disability rights provides a foundation for us to understand a current challenge for individuals with disabilities. Ableism is the unfair or prejudicial treatment of people with disabilities including children with medical complexity. It involves attitudes, practices, and societal structures that consider people with disabilities as inferior and can occur during healthcare encounters. Ableism in healthcare poses significant risk to the health and well-being of people with disabilities. It has been associated with unequal treatment, leading to the direct denial of adequate care and indirectly to loss of trust and avoidance of care (Krnjacki et al., 2018; Moscoso-Porras & Alvarado, 2018). Unfortunately, ableism is ubiquitous throughout the healthcare system due to explicit and implicit bias (Hackett et al., 2020; Ryan & Scior, 2016; Temple et al., 2019; Uysal et al., 2014; VanPuymbrouck et al., 2020) and is engrained in our structures and systems of care which favor typically developing children (Iezzoni et al., 2021; Ma & Mak, 2022). Ableism can damage the health and well-being of children with disabilities and stifle opportunities for full participation in their communities (Moscoso-Porras & Alvarado, 2018; Pascoe & Smart Richman, 2009).

The drivers of ableism in pediatrics are multifaceted; these include physician lack of knowledge and skill in caring for people with disabilities due to limited training on disability, provider disinterest in caring for CMC due to complexity of care and time needed, and implicit biases (Ames et al., 2023; Iezzoni et al., 2021).

One significant driver is assumptions regarding quality of life and worthiness for care. More than 80% of adult physicians report people with disability as having a worse quality of life than non-disabled people (Iezzoni et al., 2021). However, many people with disabilities and families of children with disability report their quality of life to be good to excellent (Costello et al., 2015; Ellzey et al., 2015; Nolan et al., 2014). The misprediction of quality of life, referred to as the disability paradox (Albrecht & Devlieger, 1999), exemplifies a significant bias against disability and can be harmful if it influences medical decision making (Klee et al., 2022; National Council on Disability, 2019; Zhong et al., 2011). This is especially concerning when quality of life becomes conflated with futility.

Ableism presents for CMC in many ways. It can show up in interpersonal interactions in which children are dehumanized and interaction is limited (Ames et al., 2023). When bias influences a healthcare provider's clinical decision making, it can lead to radically different clinical assessments and treatment options when compared to children without medical complexity, culminating in substandard care (Ames et al., 2023; Glader & Murphy, 2024). Ableism is also present in healthcare system structures and policies. Examples include limited wheelchair ramps, absence of adult changing tables in restrooms, poorly designed parking lots, inaccessible clinic spaces, and lack of accommodations such as sign language interpreters. When wheelchair scales are lacking, CMC are predisposed to weight-based medication errors. Ableism can also be reflected in insurance coverage exclusions that limit access to appropriate and necessary health care services (Foster et al., 2019, 2021).

In addition to ableism, children with medical complexity and chronic conditions are more likely to face other forms of discrimination because of marginalizing identities (e.g., race, poverty) (Helton et al., 2023). Intersectionality is an important part of child and family experiences in healthcare which can further potentiate gaps in access to care (Houtrow et al., 2022). Addressing all forms of discrimination is critical to improve the healthcare and health outcomes of children with medical complexity.

References

Akins, R. S., Krakowiak, P., Angkustsiri, K., Hertz-Picciotto, I., & Hansen, R. L. (2014). Utilization patterns of conventional and complementary/alternative treatments in children with autism spectrum disorders and developmental disabilities in a population-based study. *Journal of Developmental & Behavioral Pediatrics, 35*(1), 1–10. https://doi.org/10.1097/dbp.0000000000000013

Albrecht, G. L., & Devlieger, P. J. (1999). The disability paradox: High quality of life against all odds. *Social Science & Medicine, 48*(8), 977–988. https://doi.org/10.1016/s0277-9536(98)00411-0

American College of Physicians. (n.d.). *Pediatric to adult care transitions initiative.* https://www.acponline.org/clinical-information/high-value-care/resources-for-clinicians/pediatric-to-adult-care-transitions-initiative

American Epilepsy Society. (n.d.). *Clinical practice tools.* https://aesnet.org/clinical-care/running-your-practice

Ames, S. G., Delaney, R. K., Houtrow, A. J., Delgado-Corcoran, C., Alvey, J., Watt, M. H., & Murphy, N. (2023). Perceived disability-based discrimination in health care for children with medical complexity. *Pediatrics, 152*(1), e2022060975. https://doi.org/10.1542/peds.2022-060975

Baugh Littlejohns, L., & Wilson, A. (2019). Strengthening complex systems for chronic disease prevention: A systematic review. *BMC Public Health, 19*(1), 729. https://doi.org/10.1186/s12889-019-7021-9

Bell, E., Wallace, T., Chouinard, I., Shevell, M., & Racine, E. (2011). Responding to requests of families for unproven interventions in neurodevelopmental disorders: Hyperbaric oxygen "treatment" and stem cell "therapy" in cerebral palsy. *Developmental Disabilities Research Reviews, 17*(1), 19–26. https://doi.org/10.1002/ddrr.134

Bush, G. H. W. (2016). Remarks of President George H. W. Bush at the Signing of the Americans with Disabilities Act of 1990. [Transcript]. In: *National Archives*. https://www.archives.gov/research/americans-with-disabilities/transcriptions/naid-6037492-remarks-by-the-president-during-ceremony-for-the-signing-of-the-americans-with-disabilities-act-of-1990.html

Center for Transition to Adult Health Care for Youth with Disabilities. (n.d.). *Moving to adult health care: A 6-part toolkit series for health care transition*. https://movingtoadulthealthcare.org/toolkits/

Chuang, J., & Kennedy, J. (2016). Decision-making and guardianship. In M. Pilapil, D. DeLaet, A. Kuo, C. Peacock, & N. Sharma (Eds.), *Care of adults with chronic conditions: A practical guide* (pp. 401–411). Springer. https://doi.org/10.1007/978-3-319-43827-6_30

Cohen, E., Kuo, D. Z., Agrawal, R., Berry, J. G., Bhagat, S. K. M., Simon, T. D., & Srivastava, R. (2011). Children with medical complexity: An emerging population for clinical and research initiatives. *Pediatrics, 127*(3), 529–538. https://doi.org/10.1542/peds.2010-0910

Coombes, R. (2007). Ashley X: A difficult moral choice. *BMJ (Clinical research ed.), 334*(7584), 72–73. https://doi.org/10.1136/bmj.39091.555856.B7

Costello, J. M., Mussatto, K., Cassedy, A., Wray, J., Mahony, L., Teele, S. A., Brown, K. L., Franklin, R. C., Wernovsky, G., & Marino, B. S. (2015). Prediction by clinicians of quality of life for children and adolescents with cardiac disease. *The Journal of Pediatrics, 166*(3), 679–83.e2. https://doi.org/10.1016/j.jpeds.2014.11.061

Ellzey, A., Valentine, K. J., Hagedorn, C., & Murphy, N. A. (2015). Parent perceptions of quality of life and healthcare satisfaction for children with medical complexity. *Journal of Pediatric Rehabilitation Medicine, 8*(2), 97–104. https://doi.org/10.3233/PRM-150323

Foster, C. C., Agrawal, R. K., & Davis, M. M. (2019). Home health care for children with medical complexity: Workforce gaps, policy, and future directions. *Health Aff (Millwood), 38*(6), 987–993. https://doi.org/10.1377/hlthaff.2018.05531

Foster, C. C., Chorniy, A., Kwon, S., Kan, K., Heard-Garris, N., & Davis, M. M. (2021). Children with special health care needs and forgone family employment. *Pediatrics, 148*(3), e2020035378. https://doi.org/10.1542/peds.2020-035378

Friedman, S. L., Kalichman, M. A., & Council on Children with Disabilities. (2014). Out-of-home placement for children and adolescents with disabilities. *Pediatrics, 134*(4), 836–846. https://doi.org/10.1542/peds.2014-2279

Gerber, D. M., & Coller, R. J. (2024). Standardizing medical complexity: Fruitful, formidable, or futile? *Pediatrics, 153*(6), e2023065014. https://doi.org/10.1542/peds.2023-065014

Glader, L., & Murphy, N. (2024). To consider the whole elephant: Finding our blind spots in caring for people with disabilities. *Developmental Medicine and Child Neurology, 66*(10), 1264–1265. https://doi.org/10.1111/dmcn.16068

Got Transition®. (n.d.). *Resources & Research – Special Populations*. https://www.gottransition.org/resources-and-research/special-populations.cfm

Grossberg, R. I. (2008). Psychoanalytic contributions to the care of medically fragile children. *Journal of Psychiatric Practice, 14*(5), 307–311. https://doi.org/10.1097/01.pra.0000336758.42437.1a

References

Gunther, D. F., & Diekema, D. S. (2006). Attenuating growth in children with profound developmental disability: A new approach to an old dilemma. *Archives of Pediatrics & Adolescent Medicine, 160*(10), 1013–1017. https://doi.org/10.1001/archpedi.160.10.1013

Hackett, R. A., Steptoe, A., Lang, R. P., & Jackson, S. E. (2020). Disability discrimination and well-being in the United Kingdom: A prospective cohort study. *BMJ Open, 10*(3), e035714. https://doi.org/10.1136/bmjopen-2019-035714

Helton, J. J., Asher BlackDeer, A., Banks, K. H., Pousson, M., & Gilbert, K. L. (2023). Racial discrimination of adolescents with special healthcare needs. *The Journal of Adolescent Health, 73*(2), 383–386. https://doi.org/10.1016/j.jadohealth.2023.02.03

Houtrow, A., Martin, A. J., Harris, D., Cejas, D., Hutson, R., Mazloomdoost, Y., & Agrawal, R. K. (2022). Health equity for children and youth with special health care needs: A vision for the future. *Pediatrics, 149*(Suppl 7), e2021056150F. https://doi.org/10.1542/peds.2021-056150F

Hurvitz, E., & Noritz, G. (2016). Responding to requests for novel/unproven alternative and complementary treatments. In P. Rosenbaum, G. M. Ronen, E. Racine, J. Johannesen, & B. Dan (Eds.), *Ethics in child health: Principles and cases in neurodisability* (pp. 143–152). Mac Keith Press.

Iezzoni, L. I., Rao, S. R., Ressalam, J., Bolcic-Jankovic, D., Agaronnik, N. D., Donelan, K., Lagu, T., & Campbell, E. G. (2021). Physicians' perceptions of people with disability and their health care. *Health Affairs, 40*(2), 297–306. https://doi.org/10.1377/hlthaff.2020.01452

Klee, K., Wilfond, B., Thomas, K., & Ridling, D. (2022). Conflicts between parents and clinicians: Tracheotomy decisions and clinical bioethics consultation. *Nursing Ethics, 29*(3), 685–695. https://doi.org/10.1177/09697330211023986

Krnjacki, L., Priest, N., Aitken, Z., Emerson, E., Llewellyn, G., King, T., & Kavanagh, A. (2018). Disability-based discrimination and health: Findings from an Australian-based population study. *Australian and New Zealand Journal of Public Health, 42*(2), 172–174. https://doi.org/10.1111/1753-6405.12735

Lach, L., & Birnbaum, R. (2016). The obligation to report child abuse or neglect is more complex than it seems. In P. Rosenbaum, G. M. Ronen, E. Racine, J. Johannesen, & B. Dan (Eds.), *Ethics in child health: Principles and cases in neurodisability* (pp. 203–214). Mac Keith Press.

Ma, G. Y. K., & Mak, W. W. S. (2022). Meta-analysis of studies on the impact of mobility disability simulation programs on attitudes toward people with disabilities and environmental in/accessibility. *PLoS One, 17*(6), e0269357. https://doi.org/10.1371/journal.pone.0269357

Moon, M., Macauley, R. C., Geis, G. M., Laventhal, N. T., Opel, D. J., Sexson, W. R., & Statter, M. B. (2019). Institutional ethics committees. *Pediatrics, 143*(5). https://doi.org/10.1542/peds.2019-0659

Moscoso-Porras, M. G., & Alvarado, G. F. (2018). Association between perceived discrimination and healthcare-seeking behavior in people with a disability. *Disability and Health Journal, 11*(1), 93–98. https://doi.org/10.1016/j.dhjo.2017.04.002

National Council on Disability. (2019). *Medical futility and disability bias: Part of the bioethics and disability series* [Report]. Washington, DC. https://www.ncd.gov/assets/uploads/reports/2019/ncd_medical_futility_report_508.pdf

National Resource Center for Supported Decision Making. (n.d.). https://supporteddecisionmaking.org/

Needelman, H., & Sweeney, D. (2016). The importance of beliefs and relationships in the decision-making process. In P. Rosenbaum, G. M. Ronen, E. Racine, J. Johannesen, & B. Dan (Eds.), *Ethics in child health: Principles and cases in neurodisability* (pp. 75–84). Mac Keith Press.

Newman, C., & Zurbrugg, E. (2016). How much is too much care? Interventions and life support in children with profound impairments and life-threatening conditions. In P. Rosenbaum, G. M. Ronen, E. Racine, J. Johannesen, & B. Dan (Eds.), *Ethics in child health: Principles and cases in neurodisability* (pp. 291–302). Mac Keith Press.

Nolan, R., Luther, B., Young, P., & Murphy, N. A. (2014). Differing perceptions regarding quality of life and inpatient treatment goals for children with severe disabilities. *Academic Pediatrics, 14*(6), 574–580. https://doi.org/10.1016/j.acap.2014.02.012

Pascoe, E. A., & Smart Richman, L. (2009). Perceived discrimination and health: A meta-analytic review. *Psychological Bulletin, 135*(4), 531–554. https://doi.org/10.1037/a0016059

Phoenix, M. (2016). Service provision for hard-to-reach families: What are our responsibilities? In P. Rosenbaum, G. M. Ronen, E. Racine, J. Johannesen, & B. Dan (Eds.), *Ethics in child health: Principles and cases in neurodisability* (pp. 193–201). Mac Keith Press.

Racine, E. (2016). Can moral problems of everyday clinical practice ever be resolved? A proposal for integrative pragmatist approaches. In P. Rosenbaum, G. M. Ronen, E. Racine, J. Johannesen, & B. Dan (Eds.), *Ethics in child health: Principles and cases in neurodisability* (pp. 33–48). Mac Keith Press.

Rosenbaum, P., & Gorter, J. W. (2012). The 'F-words' in childhood disability: I swear this is how we should think! *Child: Care, Health and Development, 38*(4), 457–463. https://doi.org/10.1111/j.1365-2214.2011.01338.x

Rosenbaum, P., Ronen, G. M., & Cunnigham, B. (2016). Present-day health and neurodevelopmental disability. In P. Rosenbaum, G. M. Ronen, E. Racine, J. Johannesen, & B. Dan (Eds.), *Ethics in child health: Principles and cases in neurodisability* (pp. 17–31). Mac Keith Press.

Ryan, T. A., & Scior, K. (2016). Medical students' attitudes towards health care for people with intellectual disabilities: A qualitative study. *Journal of Applied Research in Intellectual Disabilities, 29*(6), 508–518. https://doi.org/10.1111/jar.12206

Spina Bifida Association. (2023). *Transition guideline*. https://www.spinabifidaassociation.org/resource/transition.

Sufian, B., Passamano, J., & Sopchak, A. (2018). Legal issues: Guardianship and supportive decision making. In A. Hergenroeder & C. Wiemann (Eds.), *Health care transition* (pp. 293–299). Springer. https://doi.org/10.1007/978-3-319-72868-1_30

Temple, J. B., Kelaher, M., & Williams, R. (2019). Disability discrimination and avoidance in later life: Prevalence, disability differentials and association with mental health. *International Psychogeriatrics, 31*(9), 1319–1329. https://doi.org/10.1017/S1041610218001722

Temple University Institute on Disabilities. (n.d.). *Disability rights timeline*. https://disabilities.temple.edu/resources/disability-rights-timeline

Turchi, R. M., Kuo, D. Z., Rusher, J. W., Seltzer, R. R., Lehmann, C. U., Grout, R. W., & Council on Children with Disabilities, & Committee on Medical Liability and Risk Management. (2024). Considerations for alternative decision-making when transitioning to adulthood for youth with intellectual and developmental disabilities: Policy statement. *Pediatrics, 153*(6), e2024066841. https://doi.org/10.1542/peds.2024-066841

United Nations. (1989). *Convention on the rights of the child*. https://www.ohchr.org/en/instruments-mechanisms/instruments/convention-rights-child

Uysal, A., Albayrak, B., Koçulu, B., Kan, F., & Aydın, T. (2014). Attitudes of nursing students toward people with disabilities. *Nurse Education Today, 34*(5), 878–884. https://doi.org/10.1016/j.nedt.2013.09.001

Vanderbilt Kennedy Center for Research on Human Development. (n.d.). *Health care for adults with intellectual and developmental disabilities: Toolkit for primary care providers*. https://iddtoolkit.vkcsites.org/

VanPuymbrouck, L., Friedman, C., & Feldner, H. (2020). Explicit and implicit disability attitudes of healthcare providers. *Rehabilitation Psychology, 65*(2), 101–112. https://doi.org/10.1037/rep0000317

Varkey, B. (2021). Principles of clinical ethics and their application to practice. *Medical Principles and Practice, 30*(1), 17–28. https://doi.org/10.1159/000509119

World Health Organization (WHO). (2002). *Towards a common language for functioning, disability and health: ICF* [Report]. https://www.who.int/publications/m/item/icf-beginner-s-guide-towards-a-common-language-for-functioning-disability-and-health

References

Yu, J. A., McKernan, G., Hagerman, T., Schenker, Y., & Houtrow, A. (2021). Most children with medical complexity do not receive care in well-functioning health care systems. *Hospital Pediatrics, 11*(2), 183–191. https://doi.org/10.1542/hpeds.2020-0182

Zhong, R., Knobe, J., Feigenson, N., & Mercurio, M. R. (2011). Age and disability biases in pediatric resuscitation among future physicians. *Clinical Pediatrics, 50*(11), 1001–1004. https://doi.org/10.1177/0009922811410053

Chapter 5
Implications for Policy and Practice

Introduction

In its landmark 2001 report, "**Crossing the Quality Chasm: A New Health System for the 21st Century,**" the Institute of Medicine (now the National Academy of Medicine) highlighted the significant gap between the health care that people receive and the health care that is possible with current medical knowledge and technology. It called for a comprehensive redesign of the American healthcare system to bridge this gap. The report outlined six key aims for improvement in health care:

1. **Safety**: Reducing harm caused by medical errors.
2. **Effectiveness**: Providing services based on scientific knowledge to all who could benefit.
3. **Patient-Centeredness**: Ensuring that care is respectful of and responsive to individual patient preferences, needs, and values.
4. **Timeliness**: Reducing waits and sometimes harmful delays for both those who receive and those who give care.
5. **Efficiency**: Avoiding waste, including waste of equipment, supplies, ideas, and energy.
6. **Equity**: Providing care that does not vary in quality because of personal characteristics such as gender, ethnicity, geographic location, and socioeconomic status (Institute of Medicine, 2001).

These principles aim to guide policymakers, healthcare leaders, clinicians, and other stakeholders in improving the quality of health care in the United States. The report proposed 10 rules to follow to obtain a better twenty-first century healthcare system; among other things, these include care being based on continuous healing relationships, care customized according to patient's needs and values, having the patient be the source of control, free flow of information, evidence-based decision making, making safety a system priority, decreasing waste, and cooperation among clinicians (Institute of Medicine, 2001).

The report suggested that health systems should organize around priority conditions. Priority conditions were defined using criteria including prevalence, burden of illness, cost, variability in practice, and the potential to improve value of care. While not explicitly listed in the report as a priority condition, it was clear to those caring for children with medical complexity (CMC) that this population was and remains a priority condition.

When the report was released in 2001, it was clear that care for CMC stood on the wrong side of this quality chasm. Care was generally fragmented between multiple specialists with variable input from primary care providers and poor communication between the many clinicians involved. Ancillary services were variable and often segregated from other clinical care providers. Decision making was often very prescriptive and did not always involve the parent or patient in shared decision making. Procedures were frequently done based on what could be done and not necessarily on what should be done. Oftentimes, functional outcomes and quality of life were secondary in decision making. This led to situations where a CMC may not be receiving adequate care in some areas and/or experience over-medicalization in others. Payment systems were fee-for-service based, with little correlation to the actual time and effort it took to take care of this population. CMC as a population were often lumped into children with special health care needs (CSHCN) regarding population-based data collection and outcomes, which made evaluation of the significance and scope of the population difficult.

In the more than two decades since this report was published, how far have we come toward crossing that quality chasm? There have certainly been improvements. CMC are defined by mostly universally accepted criteria, which allows descriptive data and value improvement work to proceed. Many payment models now recognize some of the non-face-to-face time commitment required to care for this population. Communication among providers is improved. Most importantly, with the emergence of specialty centers designed to optimize the treatment of CMC, many standards of care, including shared decision making, prioritizing functional outcomes, and improved overall value of care, are emerging.

This chapter serves as a summary of how elements of policy and practice contribute to our joint journey to cross the quality chasm.

Definition of Children with Medical Complexity

Any discussion of the implications of policy and practice on the financial considerations of the care for CMC requires a consistent definition of who those children are. Historically, many descriptions of this group were complicated by the inclusion of children with less complex but chronic conditions such as type 1 diabetes, attention deficit hyperactivity disorder, or asthma in the context of an otherwise well child. Furthermore, the inclusion of children with special health care needs, which is a much larger, albeit less financially impactful group, has also muddied the water. Fortunately, over the past 10 to 15 years, a consensus definition for CMC has emerged. For the purposes of our discussion, children with medical complexity share four key characteristics:

1. **Multiple chronic conditions.** An underlying disorder or set of disorders causes chronic disease in three or more body systems and requires subspecialty level care. These three conditions could be complications of one underlying diagnosis or multiple separate diagnoses.
2. **Functional limitations**: CMC often face significant functional impacts related to their underlying disorder. These functional impacts require additional treatments and therapeutic inputs to maximize participation and function.
3. **High healthcare needs.** CMC require frequent intensive healthcare services. These may include hospitalizations, specialty visits, expensive therapeutics, and durable medical equipment.
4. **Medical technology dependencies.** Many CMC rely on medical devices such as gastrostomy tubes, tracheostomy, ventilators, mobility aids, etc. to maintain quality of life, maximize functional ability, and maintain health (Cohen et al., 2011).

Multiple algorithms have been designed and validated to help identify CMC within population-based datasets. In Feudtner's Chronic Complex Condition (CCC) System, children are assessed for the presence or absence of one or more CCCs in each of 10 body systems. Additional modifiers are applied for technology dependency and/or history of transplantation (Feinstein et al., 2024). This algorithm was originally designed to assess mortality risk among populations of children with chronic diagnoses. The Pediatric Medical Complexity Algorithm (PMCA) was developed to describe complexity and chronicity of illness and stratified children by level of medical complexity. This validated algorithm has been used to assess differences in levels of care across levels of complexity in CMC (Simon et al., 2017). The Children with Disabilities Algorithm (CWD) uses ICD9/10 codes to identify children with disabilities which is an independent but intersecting group of children with chronic diagnosis (Chien et al., 2015). Lastly, the 3M™ Clinical Risk Grouping (CRG) algorithm is a commercially available tool designed to assess care cost and utilization and to predict future utilization and needs (Low et al., 2018).

Demographics

Applying the consensus definition to the National Survey of Children's Health 2016–2017 data set, 1.5% of children in the sample were classified as CMC, representing nearly 1.2 million children in the United States (Yu et al., 2021). In this cohort, CMC status was significantly associated with male sex, minority race or ethnicity, and socioeconomic adversity (Cohen et al., 2012). In our complex care program, a majority of patients had 3–5 organ systems involved in their disorder, with neurologic, gastrointestinal, and congenital/genetic CCC categories being the most common (Alvey et al., 2019). A study of 1.9 million children from Colorado, Massachusetts, and New Hampshire showed that anywhere from 0.7% to 11.4% fit criteria for medical complexity depending on the algorithm and coding criteria applied (Leyenaar et al., 2022). In this study, 48.4% of the children were female, 87.8% resided in urban areas, and 45.1% had government sponsored insurance as their only primary payer. CMC had significantly greater odds of mortality with an adjusted odds ratio of 9.97 (95% CI, 7.70–12.89) and increased utilization of health care services with an adjusted odds ratio of 4.59 (95% CI, 4.44–4.73) (Leyenaar et al., 2022).

Direct Healthcare Costs

The 1.5% of children who fit the definition of CMC incur a disproportionate amount of direct healthcare expenditure. This is not only due to episodic illnesses and exacerbations of chronic conditions, but also due to reliance on expensive equipment, procedures, medications, and ancillary care to maintain health and function. These children require services from ambulatory, primary care, inpatient, and ancillary providers at a very frequent cadence. CMC account for approximately 30–33% of total pediatric healthcare costs, 56% of hospitalizations, 39–82% of hospital days, and 53–86% of hospital charges in US children's hospitals (Murphy et al., 2020; Berry et al., 2013, 2014; Neff et al., 2004).

Indirect Healthcare Costs

Along with documented direct costs of care, families face stressors from indirect costs of caring for CMC. By some estimates, as many as 80% of families reported experiencing at least one hardship, with ~70% of families reporting financial hardship and ~50% reporting social hardship (Thomson et al., 2016; Kuo et al., 2011). An analysis of families of 324,323 CMC reported that caregivers had to devote 11–20 hours/week to direct home care and 1–6 hours per week on care coordination for their CMC (Kuo et al., 2011). Additionally, 56.8% reported financial problems, 54.1% reported a family member had to stop working outside the home due to the child's health, 48.8% reported at least 1 unmet medical need and 33.1% reported difficulty in accessing nonmedical services (Kuo et al., 2011). In another study of families with CSHCN, annual lost potential earnings from foregone employment were estimated at $18,000 per family in 2016 dollars (Foster et al., 2021). Families also often pay for uncovered medications and services (Allshouse et al., 2018), with reported out-of-pocket costs over $1000 per year (Kuo et al., 2011).

Models of Care

Ambulatory

To better address the needs of CMC, multiple clinical models have been developed with the goal of improving the value of healthcare for CMC. Models include primary care medical homes, hospital-based consultative programs, disease-specific programs, transitional programs, and more. Regardless of the specific model of care, components that are required of any program caring for CMC include family-centered care with input from caregivers regarding program design, knowledge regarding chronic and complex conditions by providers and ancillary staff, system supports to maximize function and participation, and continuous quality improvement methodology. Given the wide number of care models available, many CMC participate in multiple overlapping programs simultaneously (Cohen et al., 2011).

In the medical home model, a primary care physician provides longitudinal care, acute care, and typically provides care coordination. A patient-centered primary care medical home has many components, including a multidisciplinary care team, comprehensive range of services for acute and chronic care, a patient-centered focus, a coordinated care plan, accessible care, quality and safety measures, and aims to improve value via payment reforms. In 2004, the American Academy of Pediatrics (AAP) issued care guidelines for providing care for children with cerebral palsy in a primary care medical home setting. These included recommendations for neuromotor screening, early diagnosis, coordination of care, and in-office care of common problems associated with cerebral palsy such as spasticity, feeding disorders, respiratory complications, and orthopedic complications (Cooley, 2004). A 2004 quality improvement project in Boston area practices included introduction of a pediatric nurse practitioner as a case manager, having a parent consultant to the primary care practice, development of individualized care plans, and continuing medical education for health care professionals, which led to easier delivery of care, improved access, improved goal setting, and improved patient–physician relationships. There was also a decrease in parental work absenteeism and a reduced hospitalization rate (Palfrey et al., 2004). An evaluation of 1012 children seen in a CMC-specific hospital-based primary care clinic in Colorado showed that there were no significant differences in the cost to the hospital of patients enrolled in the special primary care clinic in comparison with CMC who were not enrolled (Berman et al., 2005). However, they did note a significant decrease in average length of stay for non-intensive care hospitalizations of CMC enrolled in the clinic program (Berman et al., 2005). While CMC who receive care in a primary care medical home do report generally better access to care and better care coordination, nearly half of CMC do not have access to a primary care office that has all criteria for medical home designation. Additional barriers to this model include a lack of provider knowledge, lack of care coordination services, long distances between primary care practices and specialty centers in much of the nation, time constraints, and inadequate financial compensation for the high amount of time required to care for this population (Strickland et al., 2004).

In a consultative model, a group with specialized clinicians and ancillary resources provides episodic care over time to CMC, typically in the setting of a tertiary children's hospital. These programs often combine physicians with experience and knowledge in treating CMC, care coordinators, nurses, social work, dietitians, etc. In the first decade of our program in Utah, we noted a 15% decrease in emergency department visits, 67% increase in observation visits, 32% decrease in hospital admissions, 68% decrease in hospital length of stay, and 69% decrease in total hospital cost (Murphy et al., 2020). CMC with tracheostomy and ventilator dependencies demonstrated the most significant reductions in mean total length of stay and mean hospital costs in a pre/post analysis. 89% of parents in the program agreed or strongly agreed that they "receive exactly what I want and need, exactly when and how I want and need it" (Murphy et al., 2020).

Disease-specific programs have arisen over the past three decades to address the comprehensive needs of children with specific chronic illnesses such as leukemia, cystic fibrosis, spina bifida, and muscular dystrophy. Many of these programs operate as a subset of the above-mentioned consultative model. In these programs, patients receive the subspecialty care needed for their chronic condition but may also receive coordination of care, access to ancillary services, and sometimes even primary care services such as urgent visits, health maintenance, vaccinations, etc.

Transitional programs are primarily designed to assist in moving CMC from hospital-based care back to the community. These might include long-term acute care centers, specialized nursing facilities, or hospital-based programs with ambulatory services. At our institution, the Connector Service was designed for CMC with complex psychosocial determinants impacting their ability to transition from inpatient to home care. This program includes physicians with experience in CMC care, care coordinators, and social workers. The program provides ambulatory visits and in-home visits with enhanced access to services to address social determinants of health.

Inpatient

Although the AAP Council on Children with Disabilities has reaffirmed that the optimal place for CMC is in a home environment (Friedman et al., 2016), they also acknowledge that more complex children in areas with fewer outpatient resources may need to congregate care in settings such as a long-term acute care (LTAC) or skilled nursing facilities (SNF).

Children with new tracheostomies and ventilator (trach/vent) dependence are among the most complex patients and can spend weeks in the intensive care unit (ICU) (Cecil et al., 2024). However, many of these children could safely transition to a lower level of care once they are medically stable. Parent training, nursing care, and coordination of outpatient durable medical equipment (DME) and home health services do not require ICU-level services. Transitioning children from the ICU to inpatient teams, LTAC, or SNF decreases the cost of care and increases ICU access for more critical patients while helping patients and families get the training and resources they need for successful discharge to home. In a study of over 4000 children with new trach/vent dependence, many had at least 7 days of ICU admission during which they did not require ICU-level care (Cecil et al., 2024). Ultimately, over 50% transitioned from the ICU to inpatient services prior to discharge to home, and nearly 16% transferred to long-term care (Cecil et al., 2024). Unfortunately, LTAC and SNF resources are not available in many states, and some intermediate care facilities cannot admit children with tracheostomies. At our institution, children who have weaned to home ventilators can transfer to inpatient teams while families complete training on their care. In addition, children who are trach/vent dependent in the community can be admitted to standard inpatient units if they are stable from a respiratory setting, avoiding ICU stays for surgeries, trauma, or non-respiratory infections.

For all CMC, lack of home health nursing can delay hospital discharge to home, adding millions of dollars of medical costs (Maynard et al., 2019; Sobotka et al., 2019). It also can lead to rehospitalization due to lack of family support and nursing expertise (Sobotka et al., 2020). Additional barriers that may cause a child to be unable to discharge to home include lack of two adults who can train on their technology or lack of outpatient DME support for home ventilators and tracheostomy supplies. With the recent recall of Respironics Trilogy ventilators, ventilator shortages also continue to complicate home discharge (Agarwal et al., 2024b). Transition through LTAC or SNF not only decreases cost and frees up hospital beds, it provides a safe environment for CMC when home resources are not available and can increase quality of life for the child and their family by getting closer to a community setting.

In the SNF environment, children can receive skilled therapy interventions and ventilator weaning in a less-restrictive environment. Families can visit to promote bonding, and children can have unlimited day visits out-of-house and up to 12 overnight visits a year. Preschool children may engage with Early Intervention programs, and school-aged children from ages 3 to 22 may attend community public schools.

Since changes to Medicaid allowing for reimbursement for SNF patients were enacted in 2018, patients admitted to SNF have become increasingly more complex. In our own experience providing pediatric care to the only two pediatric SNF in the Intermountain area, over 95% of our SNF patients are dependent on tracheostomy, most of whom are also ventilated at least 12 hours a day. We have also found that children who are admitted to SNF often have failed attempts at discharge to home, and many have failed foster care placement due to their medical fragility. Admissions to SNF can last months or years, especially for children who have trach/vent dependence. Children with neuromuscular disease, traumatic brain injury or spinal cord injuries, or genetic conditions may require invasive ventilation throughout their lives. Families may care for these children in the home for many years, but as parents age and children grow, families may no longer be able to meet their children's needs at home, and SNF services become a critical resource for ongoing long-term care.

For children dependent on ICU ventilators, inpatient and SNF services are not an option until they can transition to a home ventilator. Once these children are otherwise medically stable, however, they could transition from the ICU to long-term acute care (LTAC), which serves children on ICU ventilators. This not only decreases the cost of care, but also keeps ICU beds available for critically ill children.

LTAC facilities generally have a hospital license and are for more complicated patients with recent ICU admissions. Typical lengths of stay are 1–3 months, though some children may require several months to wean off ICU ventilators. LTAC is usually staffed by physicians with experience in pulmonary critical care. Here, children can wean to home ventilators, receive skilled therapy services, and parents can train on their care in anticipation for eventual discharge to home. In our program, complex care physicians work with subspecialty teams to identify children who are medically stable and who remain in an ICU setting only because of their requirement for an ICU ventilator. These children may then become eligible for transition of care to a pediatric-specific LTAC (Hartling et al., 2019; Kalm et al., 2021).

One subset of children for whom LTAC transition may be particularly appropriate is those with a history of preterm birth and bronchopulmonary dysplasia. Because these children average over 3 years of ventilator-dependence (Agarwal et al., 2024a), transitioning out of an ICU once they are more stable can open hundreds of ICU days for more critical patients.

Because LTAC patients are typically more stable and less fragile than their peers in the ICU, extended families and siblings can visit more often, allowing for more natural family interactions. If LTAC graduates are still unable to access sufficient outpatient services, they can transition to SNF for ongoing care.

Models of Payment

The high and rising cost of providing care for children with medical complexity places a disproportionate burden on the health care system. To address this, many systems are developing and evaluating novel models of payment for this population.

Many systems that care for CMC do so primarily in a fee-for-service environment. This traditional payment model advantages high volume low complexity conditions and procedures, which is specifically the opposite of what CMC need in their care. CMC visits are typically prolonged, require the input of multiple ancillary providers, and require extensive indirect care and care coordination provided outside of the face-to-face encounter. A review of 905 CMC in our program over a 2-year period showed that this non-face-to-face care occurred at a 2:1 ratio compared to direct care and was related to 60% of physician salary expense (Alvey et al., 2019). Historically, this time and its related expense have not been compensated, leading to financial strain on providers and systems that care for CMC. Ronis et al. (2019) showed that the median time spent in non-reimbursed care coordination in their program was 2.3 hours per child per month, with significantly greater time spent in the first month of participation in their program. They estimated the adjusted median cost of this time to be over $200 per CMC per month (Ronis et al., 2019). Strategies that have emerged to address this in fee-for-service systems include time-based billing, prolonged services codes, chronic care management programs, and hospital-based cost sharing.

Changes to Medicare and Medicaid guidelines now allow providers to bill for time spent on all services provided for a patient on the date of service. These additional services might include reviewing records, documentation, communication with other subspecialists, and test interpretation. Prolonged services codes such as CPT codes 99417 and 99418 can be used in addition to a traditional evaluation and management codes (e.g., CPT 99211-99215) when a physician or other qualified healthcare professional provides prolonged face-to-face or non-face-to-face care on a given date of service. Preliminary data from our institution show that a combination of time-based billing and prolonged services billing can significantly increase fee-for-service revenue to better match the actual work being performed by providers who care for CMC.

In Our Experience
Indirect care, which includes all interventions that support CMC and their families outside of traditional face-to-face visits (care coordination, chart reviews, informal conversations with physician colleagues, peer reviews with payers, school and homecare communications, etc.), accounts for 67% of total care time. The provision of indirect care, attention to social determinants of health, and continuous collaborations among parents, generalists, and specialists improves the care of CMC but hasn't historically been paid for in traditional fee-for-service models of compensation. The implementation of newer ways to be reimbursed for this care will likely lead to improved access to care outside of the traditional visit.

Chronic Care Management Programs

Chronic care management (CCM) services are a form of indirect healthcare provision that are intended to help patients and their families manage their health care conditions, gain access to needed resources, and reduce overall health care costs. These services include a structured recording of patient health information, maintenance of comprehensive electronic care plans, management of care transitions and other care management services, and the coordination and sharing of patient health information between providers within a system and those external to the system. Beginning in 2015, the Centers for Medicare and Medicaid Services (CMS) began paying for CCM services separately under the Physician Fee Schedule. Requirements for participation in CCM include having a continuous patient relationship with the

CMC, supporting the CMC in achieving health goals, 24/7 patient access to care and health information, preventative care, and prompt sharing of patient health information. To be eligible for CCM services, a CMC must have two or more chronic conditions that are expected to last at least 12 months or until the patient's death. These conditions must be significant enough in severity to increase the risk of death, acute exacerbation or decompensation, or functional decline. The services are not face-to-face, and eligible practitioners must bill at least 20 minutes monthly to be eligible. Eligible billing providers can include physicians, physician assistants, nurse practitioners, clinical nurse specialists, and certified nurse midwives. Clinical staff can bill for CCM under the direction of a billing practitioner on an "incident to" basis. To engage in CCM services, an initiating visit with the eligible provider must take place. This initiating visit could be during a problem-focused visit, an annual well check, or an initial intake visit. The initiating visit can be done in either the inpatient or ambulatory setting. At that visit, a provider must discuss the elements and goals of CCM, and the patient must either verbally or in writing consent to CCM services. Included in that consent should be a discussion of possible financial cost sharing responsibilities of the patient and family, the institution's availability of CCM services, and an explanation that although multiple providers could provide CCM services in a given month, only one provider may bill for those services. The initiating provider needs to document in the medical record whether the patient accepted or declined these services. Patient consent only needs to be obtained once unless the patient withdraws or changes CCM providers.

Upon completion of the initiating visit, description of CCM services, and patient consent, a comprehensive care plan needs to be created and entered into the electronic health record. This comprehensive care plan should include all health issues with a focus on chronic conditions. Elements of the comprehensive care plan should include the medical, cognitive, functional, psychosocial, and environmental aspects of the patient's condition. Specific elements would include but are not limited to a chronic problem list, expected outcomes, measurable treatment goals, functional assessment, symptom management, treatments and interventions, social determinants of health evaluation, diagnostic assessment, and coordinating health providers. Separate CPT codes exist for complex and non-complex CCM (See Table 5.1). Overall management decisions that require provider input will qualify as complex CCM. It's important to note that providers can only bill for complex CCM or non-complex CCM in a month, but not both. Additionally, they cannot report complex CCM and prolonged E/M services within the same calendar month. And, as noted, multiple providers cannot bill CCM for the same patient in the same month. To date, outcomes data related to CCM are limited. A recent study examining CCM for diabetes outcomes did find both a positive return on investment (ROI) in time spent on CCM related to revenue gained and cost savings potential related to overall reduction of A1c levels at the healthcare system level (Aguiniga et al., 2024). Another study on the implementation of CCM for patients with diabetes found more outpatient visits and fewer inpatient admissions and emergency department (ED) utilization within its population (Hong et al., 2024).

Models of Payment 79

Table 5.1 CPT Codes for Chronic Care Management Services

Code	Description
99437	Chronic care management services with the following required elements:
	− multiple (two or more) chronic conditions expected to last at least 12 months, or until the death of the patient − chronic conditions that place the patient at significant risk of death, acute exacerbation/decompensation, or functional decline − comprehensive care plan established, implemented, revised, or monitored − each additional 30 minutes by a physician or other qualified healthcare professional, per calendar month (List separately in addition to code for primary procedure)
99439	Chronic care management services with the following required elements:
	− multiple (two or more) chronic conditions expected to last at least 12 months, or until the death of the patient − chronic conditions that place the patient at significant risk of death, acute exacerbation/decompensation, or functional decline − comprehensive care plan established, implemented, revised, or monitored − each additional 20 minutes of clinical staff time directed by a physician or other qualified health care professional, per calendar month (List separately in addition to code for primary procedure)
99487[a]	Complex chronic care management services with the following required elements:
	− multiple (two or more) chronic conditions expected to last at least 12 months, or until the death of the patient − chronic conditions that place the patient at significant risk of death, acute exacerbation/decompensation, or functional decline − comprehensive care plan established, implemented, revised, or monitored, moderate or high complexity medical decision making − first 60 minutes of clinical staff time directed by a physician or other qualified healthcare professional, per calendar month
99489[a]	Complex chronic care management services with the following required elements:
	− multiple (two or more) chronic conditions expected to last at least 12 months, or until the death of the patient − chronic conditions that place the patient at significant risk of death, acute exacerbation/decompensation, or functional decline − comprehensive care plan established, implemented, revised, or monitored, moderate or high complexity medical decision making − each additional 30 minutes of clinical staff time directed by a physician or other qualified health care professional, per calendar month (List separately in addition to code for primary procedure)

(continued)

Table 5.1 (continued)

Code	Description
99490[a]	Chronic care management services with the following required elements:
	– multiple (two or more) chronic conditions expected to last at least 12 months, or until the death of the patient
	– chronic conditions that place the patient at significant risk of death, acute exacerbation/decompensation, or functional decline
	– comprehensive care plan established, implemented, revised, or monitored
	– first 20 minutes of clinical staff time directed by a physician or other qualified health care professional, per calendar month
99491[b]	Chronic care management services with the following required elements:
	– multiple (two or more) chronic conditions expected to last at least 12 months, or until the death of the patient
	– chronic conditions that place the patient at significant risk of death, acute exacerbation/decompensation, or functional decline
	– comprehensive care plan established, implemented, revised, or monitored
	– first 30 minutes provided personally by a physician or other qualified health care professional, per calendar month

[a]Includes time spent directly by the billing practitioners or clinical staff
[b]Includes time spent personally by the billing practitioner; clinical staff time does not count toward time threshold
Adapted from "Chronic Care Management Services" by Centers for Medicare and Medicaid Services, 2024a, *Medicare Learning Network Booklet 909188*, pp. 9-10, (https://www.cms.gov/outreach-and-education/medicare-learning-network-mln/mlnproducts/downloads/chroniccare-management.pdf)

Funds Flow Models

In terms of funding care for CMC within a pediatric system for both inpatient and ambulatory care, it is important to understand that CMC are a patient population that is not revenue generating. That is to say that the reimbursement received to care for this patient population does not cover the overall cost required to do so. This is not uncommon, as often there are only a few revenue-generating specialties within pediatric settings that then need to redistribute that funding surplus to cover the cost or "subsidize" those specialties that don't generate revenue to cover their costs of providing care. This results in "funds flow" models that can vary based on the financial status, size, religious affiliation, etc. of the hospital (Lakshminrusimha et al., 2022). Not all institutions accept and care for Medicaid patients, but for those that do there are often federal and state level mechanisms to help offset this burden. Whereas in an adult care setting there are multiple federal and state funding streams through CMS, in the pediatric care setting this is more limited. One mechanism is the Children's Hospital Graduate Medical Education (CHGME) program that provides some funding at the federal level to those institutions that care for Medicaid patients. In this model there is revenue associated with providing training opportunities for residents and fellows. Of note, this is funded through discretionary federal funds that can vary annually, whereas in adult settings there are more consistent appropriated funds that are pre-established and not subject to annual adjustments

(Coughlin et al., 2023). Another mechanism is a Medicaid subsidy or "match" program where states provide additional funding above and beyond the fee-for-service Medicaid rates in that state to assist in offsetting the gap that exists between the fee-for-service Medicaid dollars received for providing care and the total cost of caring for this patient population (Kusma et al., 2023). This funding typically doesn't cover the overall cost of providing care for patients, which further necessitates the need for departmental funds flow to cover the deficit that still exists. In addition, there is commonly a gap between the cost of the care coordination needed to actively manage this patient population compared to the funds provided at the institutional level, as care coordination efforts in general do not provide enough revenue-generating opportunities to cover their costs.

Accountable Care Organizations

While Accountable Care Organizations (ACOs) have been highlighted as a cost savings model since the inception of the Patient Protection and Affordable Care Act (ACA), ACOs are not a new concept in healthcare. Managed care in the United States has been identified for decades as a way to potentially simultaneously improve quality while reducing cost. ACOs are strategically designed to include quality metrics that ideally identify cost savings that can be used to fund other areas of care for the organization. Common examples of these quality metrics in pediatrics include vaccination rates, preventive care visits, and appropriate management of common conditions such as asthma, as well as reduction of high-cost point-of-care areas like emergency departments. States vary in terms of the robustness of implementation. Some states have introduced only potential upside savings for ACOs while other states have plans that are simultaneously managing both upside savings and downside risks. States also vary in terms of how these savings can be allocated, with some states requiring a certain percentage of savings to be returned to further investment by the ACO for its members.

A 2017 analysis of state Medicaid ACOs compared performance in Oregon and Colorado (McConnell et al., 2017). In both states, as in many others, states invested in separately managed ACOs, often either by region or population density. These organizations were then tasked with managing their own care within their own budgets. In both states' models, reductions in both ED and primary care visits were seen as well as improvements in preventable hospital admissions and specific quality metrics (McConnell et al., 2017). However, there are often identified populations such as CMC that don't make sense to integrate into an ACO and remain on traditional Medicaid and continue to be managed by the state.

Additional alternative payment models such as value-based payments have not been extensively deployed specifically for CMC. In fact, CMC have often been the high expense outliers that have prevented alternative payment models from working in large systems.

> **In Our Experience**
> As population health-based payment systems emerge, the episodic, difficult-to-predict, and extreme costs that CMC generate can severely impact the value or cost goals for a given cohort of covered individuals. The Pediatric Specialty Services (PSS) program in Utah was designed to use enhanced care process models, value improvement initiatives, and subsequent sharing of reduced expenses to improve the care of children in our region. While this population-health based model worked quite well for 97% of the participants, two or three CMC with high-cost hospitalizations essentially pushed the system into financial failure. Future population health-based models will need to include provisions that take into account the unpredictable and high cost of care for CMC.

Medicaid for Children with Medical Complexity

Given the extremely high cost to provide appropriate care to children with medical complexity, many of these children are primarily or secondarily insured by Medicaid plans. CMC disproportionately impacts Medicaid systems by accounting for 6–13% of enrollees, 40% of program costs, and over 40% pediatric hospital days for Medicaid insured children (Cohen et al., 2012; Ming et al., 2022). Ongoing published and anecdotal evidence demonstrates that these proportions are increasing with time (Cohen et al., 2012; Berry et al., 2014; Bergman et al., 2020). With increasing costs and decreasing resources, novel approaches to the payment for care of CMC continue to emerge. Specific innovations reviewed here include Medicaid waiver systems and the ACE Kids Act.

Medicaid Waivers

State Medicaid waiver programs allow states to modify Medicaid eligibility requirements to provide specialized benefits to certain children including CMC. They typically include modifications to the income level criteria of Medicaid eligibility. There are a wide variety of state Medicaid waiver programs in the United States. As of this writing, there are 395 active waiver programs for conditions ranging from AIDS to substance abuse to traumatic brain injury to developmental disabilities. States often use waivers to extend coverage groups that may not otherwise qualify for Medicaid due to income or other factors, to restrict enrollees to a specific network of providers, or to respond to public health emergencies. Medicaid waivers for children with disabilities are designed to provide essential services that enable a child to live at home or in a community setting rather than in an institutional environment. They often offer coverage for personalized services tailored to the specific needs of the CMC such as in-house support, respite care, and/or specialized therapies. Many programs aid families who care for CMC with an attempt to address unique needs that arise from a child's specific rare condition. Many of these programs state specific goals related to providing services and support to allow for greater independence, community participation, and cost-effective care for CMC.

Medicaid waiver programs have wide variation in resources, services, and eligibility requirements. Two examples of waiver systems that are commonly used to provide care for CMC in the state of Utah include the Utah Medically Complex Children's Waiver which provides personal attendance services, skilled nursing, respite, and financial management services to CMC aged 0 to 19 years who meet specific scoring requirements for the enrollment period and the Utah Waiver for Technology Dependent, Medically Fragile Individuals which provides personal attendant services, skilled nursing, health aides, private duty nursing, financial management services, family support, and in-home feeding therapy services to CMC aged 0 to 20 years who meet specific scoring criteria. While these waiver services allow a greater number of children to access services that they may not otherwise be able to obtain, problems related to a shortage of skilled nursing and respite care providers as well as financial limitations which disallow many CMC from enrollment continue to be problematic.

The ACE Kids Act

The Advancing Care for Exceptional (ACE) Kids Act is a significant piece of federal legislation passed by unanimous vote by both chambers of Congress as a part of the Medicaid Services Investment and Accountability Act of 2019. The Act is aimed at improving care for children with medical complexity who are enrolled in Medicaid. Participation in the program is voluntary for both states and families and requires that individual states opt into the program and follow specific federal guidance, participating providers meet specific criteria as a medical home for CMC, and children meet eligibility requirements. To participate, a child must be under 21 years of age and have at least one chronic condition that impacts three or more organ systems in a way that affects cognitive or physical functioning and that requires medication, surgical intervention, technology dependency, and/or other ongoing treatments. Additionally, children with one life-limiting illness or a rare pediatric disease as defined by the federal Food Drug and Cosmetic Act qualify for the program (Children's Hospital Association, 2019).

States are required to opt in to participation by submitting a Medicaid state plan amendment to the US Department of Health and Human Services that reflects the statutory requirements, as well as guidance from the Centers for Medicare and Medicaid Services (CMS). States that opt to participate by creating medical homes to care for CMC are eligible for a 15% increase to their Federal Medical Assistance Percentage (FMAP) for two quarters after qualification, not to exceed a total FMAP of 90%. The Act also provides up to $5,000,000 for state planning grants related to implementation (Children's Hospital Association, 2019). Participating states may develop their own methodology for payment models including population-based, fee-for-service, or alternative payment models. States are required to create methods to notify the CMC's medical home of emergency department visits, create a process to educate providers and family on the availability of services, and create guidelines for access to out-of-state care when appropriate care for rare and complex diseases is unavailable in the CMC's home state. The Act additionally specifies that guidelines for the treatment and prevention of substance abuse and mental illness among CMC should be developed. Participating states are required to report to CMS on the number and characteristics of the children enrolled in the program, the type of delivery systems and payment models used, the characteristics and number of participating providers and ACE Kid's medical homes, quality improvement measures, and the extent of out-of-state involvement (Children's Hospital Association, 2019).

In 2024, the state of Utah submitted and was awarded a state planning grant for future implementation of the ACE Kids Act. Specific to Utah's planning grant is describing the process for identifying additional chronic conditions not listed by the Social Security Administration (SSA). Utah is also focused on encouraging health home providers to operate a "whole person" philosophy that includes access to the full range of services identified in ACE Kids. Upon implementation, Utah Medicaid will develop a plan to address issues regarding prevention and treatment of mental illness and substance use for this population that will include tracking reduction of spending, inpatient days, and how to use health information exchange (HIE) to accomplish this (Strohecker, 2024). The state of Utah has identified the following goals to drive research and planning activities:

1. Identification of current system gaps focusing on CMS-required elements of health home services
2. Assessment of program design
3. Evaluation of cost
4. Evaluation of policy impact
5. Identification of clearly defined outcomes pre- and post-state planning implementation (Strohecker, 2024)

A primary goal of the Act is to create collaborative partnerships between children's hospitals and community providers to increase access to patient-centered medical homes designed to serve the needs of CMC. To qualify as a medical home for CMC, providers are expected to coordinate prompt access to needed primary, specialty, surgical, and ancillary care. They must additionally coordinate out-of-state and pediatric emergency care for their patients. Additionally, they should provide access to hospice and palliative care services in states that provide such services. Medical homes should develop care plans for enrolled children that consider the needs of the child and the family across the care spectrum. These care plans should be developed in a linguistically, culturally, and geographically appropriate manner for the family of the CMC.

The ACE Kids Act represents a significant step toward better healthcare for children with complex medical needs, ensuring they receive the coordinated and comprehensive care they deserve. One limitation that should be noted is that, as mentioned previously, the current ACE Kids funding for states that opt in is an enhanced match of up to 15% upon implementation for 6 months. While this provides a short-term increase in federal funding for states' Medicaid programs, it clearly doesn't offer a long-term solution to funding the work that ACE Kids is intended to facilitate. The hope is that through the implementation grants that participating states receive, they can create and implement a program framework and payment methodology that can sustain long-term solutions to funding this enhanced work for CMC.

Toward Bridging the Quality Chasm

How have we done over the past two decades in bridging the quality chasm that existed in 2001? Over that time, we've seen the emergence of many specialty consultative programs, increased availability of patient-centered primary care medical homes, and fee-for-service payment models that try to reimburse providers for time spent providing care outside of the traditional face-to-face visit. While these have all led to some improvements in the value of care for this population, much work remains to be done. The need for this work is amplified by the fact that the number of surviving CMC and overall proportion of pediatric healthcare utilization dedicated to CMC are both increasing significantly. It could be said that the success of many of these programs in fact creates a positive feedback loop generating a higher need for programs and models of care that target CMC.

For over four decades, CMS has required states to have a Medicaid Advisory Committee (MAC) comprised of 51% or more beneficiaries and their representatives and 49% or fewer providers and their representatives. However, in response to a 2022 Request for Information (RFI), beneficiary groups report that they continue to be concerned about lack of representation and voice. Consequently, starting in 2025, CMS will require MACs to change their format and create specific Beneficiary Advisory Committees (BACs), whose members will eventually make up 25% of MAC members (CMS, 2024b). Because both providers and beneficiaries have a voice through the MAC and BAC, these are resources physicians and families of CMC can use to communicate directly with state Medicaid leaders. When we find gaps in services that affect the health of CMC, we can argue that covering these gaps makes sense morally, as doing so decreases morbidity and mortality, and economically, when the cost of coverage for outpatient services decreases the usage of high-cost hospital services.

In conclusion, effective policies and models of care for children with medical complexity are crucial in ensuring these vulnerable populations receive the comprehensive and coordinated care they need. Since 2001, when the Institute of Medicine called for a redesign of the American healthcare system to provide higher quality care, CMC have emerged as a priority group for policy and practice improvements. Given their significant impact within healthcare systems, any policies aiming to enhance the overall value of pediatric care must address the needs of CMC. The high cost of care for CMC, coupled with their medical fragility, offers fertile ground for developing higher-value care models. These improvements must adopt a system-wide approach, encompassing ambulatory, inpatient, and transitional settings. Additionally, payment models emphasizing value and outcomes over volume are essential given the immense time required for coordinating the care of CMC. Continued investment in research and policy development is essential to address the evolving needs of this population and ensure that all children, regardless of their medical complexity, have access to high-quality, equitable healthcare. With concerted efforts from policymakers, healthcare providers, and communities, we can build a more inclusive and responsive healthcare system for all.

References

Agarwal, A., Manimtim, W. M., Alexiou, S., Abman, S. H., Akangire, G., Aoyama, B. C., Austin, E. D., Baker, C. D., Bansal, M., Bauer, S. E., Cristea, A. I., Dawson, S. K., Fierro, J. L., Hayden, L. P., Henningfeld, J. K., Kaslow, J. A., Lai, K. V., Levin, J. C., McKinney, R. L., & Collaco, J. M. (2024a). Factors associated with liberation from home mechanical ventilation and tracheostomy decannulation in infants and children with severe bronchopulmonary dysplasia. *Journal of Perinatology*. Advance online publication. https://doi.org/10.1038/s41372-024-02078-z

Agarwal, A., McKinney, R. L., Baker, C. D., Nelin, L. D., & Abman, S. H. (2024b). Adapting to changing ventilator access: Impact on management of severe bronchopulmonary dysplasia in children. *Pediatric Pulmonology, 59*(6), 1803–1806. https://doi.org/10.1002/ppul.26945

Aguiniga, A., Ebert, D., Rodriguez, E., Nguyenly, A., & Wesling, M. (2024). The effect of chronic care management on diabetes-related outcomes in interprofessional care of a medically complex patient population. *Journal of the American College of Clinical Pharmacy*. Advance online publication. https://doi.org/10.1002/jac5.2024

Alvey, J. C., Valentine, K., Wilkes, J., Bardsley, T., Marty, C., Mann, K., & Murphy, N. A. (2019). Indirect care utilization among children with medical complexity. *Current Physical Medicine and Rehabilitation Reports, 7*(1), 1–5. https://doi.org/10.1007/s40141-019-0204-6

Allshouse, C., Comeau, M., Rodgers, R., & Wells, N. (2018). Families of children with medical complexity: A view from the front lines. *Pediatrics, 141*(Supplement_3), S195–S201. https://doi.org/10.1542/peds.2017-1284d

Bergman, D. A., Keller, D., Kuo, D. Z., Lerner, C., Mansour, M., Stille, C., Richardson, T., Rodean, J., & Hudak, M. (2020). Costs and use for children with medical complexity in a care management program. *Pediatrics, 145*(4), e20192401. https://doi.org/10.1542/peds.2019-2401

Berman, S., Rannie, M., Moore, L., Elias, E., Dryer, L. J., & Jones, M. D. (2005). Utilization and costs for children who have special health care needs and are enrolled in a hospital-based comprehensive primary care clinic. *Pediatrics, 115*(6), e637–e642. https://doi.org/10.1542/peds.2004-2084

Berry, J. G., Hall, M., Hall, D. E., Kuo, D. Z., Cohen, E., Agrawal, R., Mandl, K. D., Clifton, H., & Neff, J. (2013). Inpatient growth and resource use in 28 children's hospitals. *JAMA Pediatrics, 167*(2), 170. https://doi.org/10.1001/jamapediatrics.2013.432

Berry, J. G., Hall, M., Neff, J., Goodman, D., Cohen, E., Agrawal, R., Kuo, D., & Feudtner, C. (2014). Children with medical complexity and Medicaid: Spending and cost savings. *Health Affairs, 33*(12), 2199–2206. https://doi.org/10.1377/hlthaff.2014.0828

References

Cecil, C. A., Dziorny, A. C., Hall, M., Kane, J. M., Kohne, J., Olszewski, A. E., Rogerson, C. M., Slain, K. N., Toomey, V., Goodman, D. M., & Heneghan, J. A. (2024). Low-resource hospital days for children following new tracheostomy. *Pediatrics, 154*(3). https://doi.org/10.1542/peds.2023-064920

Centers for Medicare and Medicaid Services (CMS). (2024a). *Chronic care management services* (Medicare Learning Network Booklet 909188). https://www.cms.gov/outreach-and-education/medicare-learning-network-mln/mlnproducts/downloads/chroniccaremanagement.pdf

Centers for Medicare and Medicaid Services (CMS). (2024b). Medicaid program; Ensuring access to Medicaid services. *Federal Register, 89*(92), 40542–40878.

Chien, A. T., Kuhlthau, K. A., Toomey, S. L., Quinn, J. A., Houtrow, A. J., Kuo, D. Z., Okumura, M. J., Van Cleave, J. M., Johnson, C. K., Mahoney, L. L., Martin, J., Landrum, M. B., & Schuster, M. A. (2015). Development of the children with disabilities algorithm. *Pediatrics, 136*(4), e871–e878. https://doi.org/10.1542/peds.2015-0228

Children's Hospital Association. (2019). *Summary: Advancing Care for Exceptional Kids Act (Public Law No. 116-16)*. https://www.childrenshospitals.org/-/media/files/public-policy/children_with_medical_complexity/ace_kids/ace_kids_act_summary_hr1839_042319.pdf. Accessed September 20, 2024.

Cohen, E., Berry, J. G., Camacho, X., Anderson, G., Wodchis, W., & Guttmann, A. (2012). Patterns and costs of health care use of children with medical complexity. *Pediatrics, 130*(6), e1463–e1470. https://doi.org/10.1542/peds.2012-0175

Cohen, E., Kuo, D. Z., Agrawal, R., Berry, J. G., Bhagat, S. K. M., Simon, T. D., & Srivastava, R. (2011). Children with medical complexity: An emerging population for clinical and research initiatives. *Pediatrics, 127*(3), 529–538. https://doi.org/10.1542/peds.2010-0910

Cooley, W. C. (2004). Providing a primary care medical home for children and youth with cerebral palsy. *Pediatrics, 114*(4), 1106–1113. https://doi.org/10.1542/peds.2004-1409

Coughlin, C. G., Michelson, K. A., DeLong, A. J., & Stewart, A. M. (2023). Federal funding for children's hospitals: Challenges and critical shortages for pediatric care. *Pediatrics, 152*(4), e2023061714. https://doi.org/10.1542/peds.2023-061714

Feinstein, J. A., Hall, M., Davidson, A., & Feudtner, C. (2024). Pediatric Complex Chronic Condition System Version 3. *JAMA Network Open, 7*(7), e2420579. https://doi.org/10.1001/jamanetworkopen.2024.20579

Foster, C. C., Chorniy, A., Kwon, S., Kan, K., Heard-Garris, N., & Davis, M. M. (2021). Children with special health care needs and forgone family employment. *Pediatrics, 148*(3), e2020035378. https://doi.org/10.1542/peds.2020-035378

Friedman, S. L., Norwood, K. W., Jr., & Council on Children with Disabilities. (2016). Out-of-home placement for children and adolescents with disabilities-addendum: Care options for children and adolescents with disabilities and medical complexity. *Pediatrics, 138*(6), e20163216. https://doi.org/10.1542/peds.2016-3216

Hartling, C., Mann, K., Dean, R., Brinton, J., & Murphy, N. A. (2019). *Transitioning children from NICU ventilators to home ventilators via a pediatric long term acute care unit: A new pathway* [Poster]. American Academy for Cerebral Palsy and Developmental Medicine annual meeting.

Hong, D., Stoecker, C., Shao, Y., Nauman, E., Fonseca, V., Hu, G., Bazzano, A. N., Kabagambe, E. K., & Shi, L. (2024). Effects of non-face-to-face chronic care management on service utilization and outcomes among US Medicare beneficiaries with diabetes. *Journal of General Internal Medicine, 39*(11), 1985–1992. https://doi.org/10.1007/s11606-024-08667-0

Institute of Medicine Committee on Quality of Health Care in America. (2001). *Crossing the quality chasm: A new health system for the 21st century*. National Academies Press.

Kalm, B., Lai, K., & Darro, N. (2021). Care of children with home mechanical ventilation in the healthcare continuum. *Hospital Practice, 49*(Suppl 1), 456–466. https://doi.org/10.1080/21548331.2021.1988608

Kuo, D. Z., Cohen, E., Agrawal, R., Berry, J. G., & Casey, P. H. (2011). A national profile of caregiver challenges among more medically complex children with special health care needs.

Archives of Pediatrics and Adolescent Medicine, 165(11), 1020. https://doi.org/10.1001/archpediatrics.2011.172

Kusma, J. D., Raphael, J. L., Perrin, J. M., Hudak, M. L., & Committee on Child Health Financing. (2023). Medicaid and the children's health insurance program: Optimization to promote equity in child and young adult health. *Pediatrics, 152*(5), e2023064088. https://doi.org/10.1542/peds.2023-064088

Lakshminrusimha, S., Murin, S., Kirk, J. D., Mustafa, Z., Maurice, T. R., Sousa, N., Lee, J., & Lubarsky, D. A. (2022). "Funds flow" implementation at academic health centers: Unique challenges to pediatric departments. *The Journal of Pediatrics, 249*, 6–10.e4.

Leyenaar, J. K., Schaefer, A. P., Freyleue, S. D., Austin, A. M., Simon, T. D., Van Cleave, J., Moen, E. L., O'Malley, A. J., & Goodman, D. C. (2022). Prevalence of children with medical complexity and associations with health care utilization and in-hospital mortality. *JAMA Pediatrics, 176*(6), e220687. https://doi.org/10.1001/jamapediatrics.2022.0687

Low, L. L., Yan, S., Kwan, Y. H., Tan, C. S., & Thumboo, J. (2018). Assessing the validity of a data driven segmentation approach: A 4 year longitudinal study of healthcare utilization and mortality. *PLoS ONE, 13*(4), e0195243. https://doi.org/10.1371/journal.pone.0195243

Maynard, R., Christensen, E., Cady, R., Jacob, A., Ouellette, Y., Podgorski, H., Schiltz, B., Schwantes, S., & Wheeler, W. (2019). Home health care availability and discharge delays in children with medical complexity. *Pediatrics, 143*(1), e20181951. https://doi.org/10.1542/peds.2018-1951

McConnell, K. J., Renfro, S., Chan, B. K. S., Meath, T. H. A., Mendelson, A., Cohen, D., Waxmonsky, J., McCarty, D., Wallace, N., & Lindrooth, R. C. (2017). Early performance in Medicaid accountable care organizations. *JAMA Internal Medicine, 177*(4), 538. https://doi.org/10.1001/jamainternmed.2016.9098

Ming, D. Y., Jones, K. A., White, M. J., Pritchard, J. E., Hammill, B. G., Bush, C., Jackson, G. L., & Raman, S. R. (2022). Healthcare utilization for Medicaid-insured children with medical complexity: Differences by sociodemographic characteristics. *Maternal and Child Health Journal, 26*(12), 2407–2418. https://doi.org/10.1007/s10995-022-03543-x

Murphy, N. A., Alvey, J., Valentine, K. J., Mann, K., Wilkes, J., & Clark, E. B. (2020). Children with medical complexity: The 10-year experience of a single center. *Hospital Pediatrics, 10*(8), 702–708. https://doi.org/10.1542/hpeds.2020-0085

Neff, J. M., Sharp, V. L., Muldoon, J., Graham, J., & Myers, K. (2004). Profile of medical charges for children by health status group and severity level in a Washington state health plan. *Health Services Research, 39*(1), 73–90. https://doi.org/10.1111/j.1475-6773.2004.00216.x

Palfrey, J. S., Sofis, L. A., Davidson, E. J., Liu, J., Freeman, L., & Ganz, M. L. (2004). The pediatric alliance for coordinated care: Evaluation of a medical home model. *Pediatrics, 113*(Supplement_4), 1507–1516. https://doi.org/10.1542/peds.113.s4.1507

Ronis, S. D., Grossberg, R., Allen, R., Hertz, A., & Kleinman, L. C. (2019). Estimated nonreimbursed costs for care coordination for children with medical complexity. *Pediatrics, 143*(1), e20173562. https://doi.org/10.1542/peds.2017-3562

Simon, T. D., Cawthon, M. L., Popalisky, J., & Mangione-Smith, R. (2017). Development and validation of the Pediatric Medical Complexity Algorithm (PMCA) Version 2.0. *Hospital Pediatrics, 7*(7), 373–377. https://doi.org/10.1542/hpeds.2016-0173

Sobotka, S. A., Foster, C., Lynch, E., Hird-McCorry, L., & Goodman, D. M. (2019). Attributable delay of discharge for children with long-term mechanical ventilation. *The Journal of Pediatrics, 212*, 166–171. https://doi.org/10.1016/j.jpeds.2019.04.034

Sobotka, S. A., Lynch, E., Peek, M. E., & Graham, R. J. (2020). Readmission drivers for children with medical complexity: Home nursing shortages cause health crises. *Pediatric Pulmonology, 55*(6), 1474–1480. https://doi.org/10.1002/ppul.24744

Strickland, B., McPherson, M., Weissman, G., van Dyck, P., Huang, Z. J., & Newacheck, P. (2004). Access to the medical home: Results of the national survey of children with special health care needs. *Pediatrics, 113*(5 Suppl), 1485–1492.

References

Strohecker, J. (2024). *New Fiscal Year Social Services Base Budget: Health Homes for Children with Medically Complex Conditions* [Report]. Utah Department of Health and Human Services, State of Utah Division of Integrated Healthcare. https://le.utah.gov/interim/2024/pdf/00002463.pdf

Thomson, J., Shah, S. S., Simmons, J. M., Sauers-Ford, H. S., Brunswick, S., Hall, D., Kahn, R. S., & Beck, A. F. (2016). Financial and social hardships in families of children with medical complexity. *The Journal of Pediatrics, 172*, 187–193.e1. https://doi.org/10.1016/j.jpeds.2016.01.049

Yu, J. A., McKernan, G., Hagerman, T., Schenker, Y., & Houtrow, A. (2021). Identifying children with medical complexity from the national survey of children's health combined 2016-17 data set. *Hospital Pediatrics, 11*(2), 192–197. https://doi.org/10.1542/hpeds.2020-0180

Chapter 6
Looking Ahead: Children with Medical Complexity and Public Health, Workforce Training, and Advocacy

A Healthcare System Call to Action

Medicine is a dynamic, rapidly changing science. Just over 25 years ago, children with special healthcare needs (CSHCN) became a recognized pediatric population (McPherson et al., 1998). CSHCN are now a well-recognized and well-understood group of children, accounting for 19% of the US pediatric population (Health Resources & Services Administration, 2022). In the last 10–15 years, we have seen a subpopulation of CSHCN emerge. Children with the highest levels of medical complexity, medical fragility, technology dependencies, and functional limitations are now surviving and thriving. Historically, such children would have survived only in hospitals and died early in childhood from their life-limiting conditions. Yet, innovative medical interventions, advanced home-based technologies, and community-based resources now support this growing population. In 2011, we came to recognize this small and impactful group as children with medical complexity (CMC) (Cohen et al., 2011). Currently, it is estimated that CMC account for 1–2% of the US pediatric population (Yu et al., 2021).

In the previous chapters, we described the current state of the art in health care for CMC, including advances in care delivery as well as the inherent limitations and challenges. Looking into the next decade or two, we can imagine that CMC will account for far more than 1% of the pediatric population. Innovative gene therapies continue to transform previously lethal neuromuscular disorders into chronic complex conditions. Similarly, enzyme replacement therapies for children with metabolic disorders and complex congenital heart surgeries for infants with trisomy 13 and trisomy 18 are changing the trajectories of these conditions. We are responsible for the delivery of high value, accessible, and continuous care for increasing numbers of CMC and their families, in pace with the development of life-sustaining interventions. And as we celebrate the growing numbers of CMC who become adults with medical complexity and chronic complex conditions, we are similarly called to care for them in adult healthcare systems.

In this chapter, we apply our individual and collective experiences and the lessons learned over the past two decades to envision a brighter future for CMC and their families. Our vision is that healthcare systems, public policies, and community programs adapt and expand to meet the multifaceted needs of CMC and their families. And at the same time, CMC and their families enrich our professional fulfillment by advancing our intellectual, ethical, moral, and cultural experiences of care. They remind us that humanism, kindness, and community are the reasons that we all invest in the public health of caring.

A Well-Prepared Pediatric Workforce

We need a well-prepared and sufficiently large pediatric workforce to care for the growing population of CMC. By 2032, major workforce shortages in the primary care disciplines and in many specialties are expected (Vinci, 2021). Almost 50% of children's hospitals report vacancies in developmental and behavioral pediatrics and adolescent and child psychiatry, and more than 30% of children's hospitals report vacancies in child neurology and genetics (Vinci, 2021). Similarly, the physical medicine and rehabilitation (PM&R) workforce will continue to have a national shortfall of more than 10% in 2030 (Dall et al., 2021). The subspeciality of pediatric rehabilitation medicine (PRM), with focused expertise on caring for children with disabilities, is limited by training requirements and a lack of standards regarding the core knowledge, skills, and attitudes of PRM providers (Turk et al., 2023). Academicians debate the value of proposing a new pediatric subspecialty of complex care, particularly given the overlapping of expertise with multiple subspecialties. The rapidly expanding scope of complex care pediatrics challenges standardization of entrustable professional activities (EPAs) for complex care pediatricians.

> **In Our Experience**
> In 2007, Edward Clark, MD, Chair of the Department of Pediatrics, recognized the need for a system of care for the children in our region with the highest levels of medical complexity, fragility, technology dependencies, and functional limitations. He envisioned a value-based system of population health. We got started and learned along the way. The Comprehensive Care program was solidly in place by 2011, at the same time that the complex pediatric population was nationally recognized as CMC. In 2018, Angelo Giardino, MD, PhD, accepted the baton as department chair and carried forward the support for and investment in complex care pediatrics. We are indebted to the visionary leadership of Dr. Clark and Dr. Giardino, prioritizing the care of CMC and their families through high functioning health care systems and investing in future generations of well-prepared pediatric providers.

The occupational phenomenon of burnout, amplified by the COVID-19 pandemic, is well documented among healthcare providers. For pediatricians, burnout may relate to the character traits that attract trainees to the field, namely, compassion and altruism. Moreover, caring for children who are chronically ill and/or medically vulnerable can exacerbate compassion fatigue, emotional exhaustion, and moral distress (McClafferty, 2024). Nationally, women physicians have higher rates of burnout as compared to men. With women accounting for 73% of the pediatric physician workforce (American Board of Pediatrics, 2024), attention to the pediatric physician workforce is urgently needed. In a recent cross-sectional study of academic physicians, 33% indicate an intention to leave their current positions within 2 years, citing reasons of burnout, lack of professional fulfillment, and issues of well-being (Ligibel et al., 2023). Comprehensive approaches to reduce physician turnover are critical. Shanafelt (2021) reminds us that the last three decades have a been a time of tremendous progress for the field of physician well-being, moving from an era of distress, characterized by ignorance and neglect, to an era of awareness and insight. This progress should be invested in developing a physician workforce that is strong, healthy, and sustainable.

Pediatric residents feel overwhelmed when caring for CMC (Bogetz et al., 2014, 2015). They encounter multifaceted challenges, including a lack of "ownership" for patients, limited decision-making authority, restricted autonomy, and insufficient care coordination resources to address the extensive psychosocial needs of CMC. Residents also struggle when multiple specialists offer disparate recommendations ("too many cooks in the kitchen"). Integrating principles of shared decision making and promoting longitudinal relationships with CMC and their families into pediatric residencies are proposed solutions. Additionally, faculty educators can support resident education by openly discussing their own challenges in caring for CMC with trainees, cultivating humility amongst learners and faculty.

To ensure a well-prepared pediatric workforce, we must recruit well-qualified medical students into pediatric residencies and subspecialty training programs, and then empower them with the knowledge, skills, and attitudes that best support the care of CMC and their families across the lifespan. Currently, there are no established competencies from the Accreditation Council for Graduate Medical Education regarding care for CMC, and only a third of pediatric residency programs have specific CMC curricula for their trainees (Sieplinga et al., 2023). An alarming number of pediatric residents do not feel confident in key areas of caring for CMC (Murphy Salem et al., 2022). Pediatric residents from a large academic center were surveyed regarding their confidence level in performing skills required to care for CMC. While trainees had modest increases in confidence as they progressed through residency, the responses indicated that, on average, the residents (even those about to graduate) felt only slightly to somewhat confident in these skills on a 5-point Likert scale ranging from "Not at all" to "Extremely" (Murphy Salem et al., 2022).

> **In Our Experience**
> Complex care pediatrics is just beginning to offer post graduate training programs and novel non-accredited fellowships. Our current model at the University of Utah Department of Pediatrics is that of a 12-month "clinical instructorship" that offers dedicated time and education for pediatricians to become proficient complex care providers. The curriculum is a potpourri of general and subspecialist experiences across the continuum in a major academic health center. Our inaugural "fellow" (EAH) is now an assistant professor, contributing greatly to the future workforce and scholarly endeavors that advance the field.

Pediatric residents need training programs that develop their competence and confidence in caring for CMC. Didactic sessions, interactive cased-based discussions, hands-on simulations, community-based experiences, and rich clinical experiences are among the essential educational elements. Families of CMC can also contribute to the education, sharing their lived experiences and personal stories that contribute to the capability and confidence of the next generation of complex care pediatricians.

Strong and Steady Pediatric Advocacy

Families as Providers, Educators, and Advocates

We need to listen to and learn from families of CMC. These families report poor outcomes related to their own emotional well-being, family functioning, and financial stability (Yu et al., 2022). Screeners that identify social determinants of health for CMC and their families can open conversations that lead to more resources and better outcomes. Families and providers seek to address the pervasive disability-based discrimination (ableism) that strains access to care (Ames et al., 2023; Allshouse et al., 2018), by upholding principles of human dignity, creativity, and trusted partnerships (Houlihan et al., 2024). As discussed in Chap. 4, the four pillars of medical ethics (beneficence, nonmaleficence, autonomy, and justice) provide a solid foundation for healthcare partnerships that optimize outcomes for CMC and families.

Parents and family caregivers are key members of their child's healthcare teams. We count on them to regularly assess their child's health, administer complex medication and feeding regimens, continuously manage medical technologies, and be available 24/7 to respond to acute illnesses and, not infrequently, urgencies and emergencies. As parents are essential healthcare workers for their children, they need trusted and skilled respite services that sustain them. As described in Chap. 3, home health care, in-home and community-based programs, and waivers that pay family members for their skilled work offer novel approaches to an unmet need yet vary state to state.

> **In Our Experience**
> As part of our pediatric residency program's advocacy training, second-year residents rotate with complex care faculty and staff in outpatient clinics and post-acute care community sites. They learn firsthand of the daily experiences of CMC and their families, explore available resources for families that support care at home, and identify advocacy opportunities. Upon completion, residents report increased levels of respect for and less fear of CMC and their families; some even adjust their career plans to include the care of CMC.

Pediatricians as Legislative Advocates

The American Academy of Pediatrics (AAP) Curriculum Committee includes advocacy training as a core pediatric residency competency. AAP chapters are key stakeholders in pediatric advocacy, described as "an integral part of the professional role and duty of the pediatrician" (Rushton & AAP Committee on Community Health Services, 2005). The AAP offers Community Access to Child Health (CATCH) grants to empower residents in identifying and addressing gaps in child health services through community action. Residents who participate in project-based and community-based advocacy are more likely to continue participating in advocacy throughout their careers (Goldshore et al., 2014). Additionally, senior residents who mentor their junior peers ensure that an advocacy project is maintained for several subsequent years (Anderson et al., 2024).

Pediatricians and pediatric trainees can advocate through state and national medical associations. In the United States, both the state associations and the American Medical Association have their own House of Delegates, which acts as the legislative and policy-making body of the organizations. Delegates are comprised of medical students, residents, and practicing physicians. Pediatric delegates can craft resolutions that address children's health issues. Working together with specialty organizations and state and national medical organizations, pediatricians can amplify messages that support access to high-quality healthcare services. Encouraging our pediatric trainees to get involved can position them to become powerful advocates for children throughout their careers.

> **In Our Experience**
> In the Utah Chapter of the AAP, medical student and resident representatives join the chapter's leaders in setting local and regional priorities. During annual state legislative seasons, pediatricians and trainees meet policy makers, build relationships with their individual elected representatives, testify in committees, and learn more about the legislative process. In addition to state level advocacy, pediatricians and pediatric residents can serve as delegates to the national AAP Leadership Conference, influencing new policy to support children's healthcare.

Advocacy with Payers, Policy Makers, and Community Stakeholders

Over the past decade, models of provider compensation for direct and indirect care rendered in primary care medical homes, consultative complex care programs, and hospitals have evolved (See Chap. 5). Value-based approaches for populations of CMC are needed to connect traditional medical services with community programs. Integrated systems that support home and community-based care rather than high-cost, crisis-driven acute care hospitalizations for CMC offer the greatest potential for high-value care. While we continue to first think of children's hospitals and clinics when considering health care delivery for CMC, the home and community settings are where most children receive their daily medical care (Foster et al., 2025). Home health care is an essential and under-recognized, under-resourced, under-valued provider of services, equipment, and supplies in a child's home and community. Continued investment in research, policy and program implementation is essential to address the evolving needs of CMC across the public health continuum. With concerted efforts from policymakers, healthcare providers, and communities, we envision a more inclusive and responsive healthcare system for all.

Summary and Future Directions

The good news is that we are making progress. We now know that CMC are a small, rapidly growing, and meaningful pediatric population. We are convinced that healthcare systems designed for typically developing children cannot meet the needs of CMC and their families. We agree that partnerships with all stakeholders can improve outcomes. Parents of CMC inspire us with their deep dedication to and joy in caring for their CMC. Medical educators are better preparing future pediatricians to care for CMC, with an increased awareness of individual cultures, values, and goals, and in alignment with families and communities. We are investing nationally in provider well-being and professional fulfillment, replacing burnout with a renewed experience of joy in medicine.

Yet, we still have much to do. On the strong foundation of the past two decades (disability rights, medical ethics, medical science and education, healthcare policy, public health programs), we must further advance health and community systems of care for CMC and their families. High quality medical care without high functioning systems of public and community health is of limited benefit. We need to address social determinants of health with strong public health programs. The future of complex care pediatrics depends on the integration of basic and applied clinical sciences, healthcare delivery practices, family and community systems, health policy frameworks, public health processes, and a big gulp of humble pie. While we envision a perfect system of care, we are also called to be present, to expect the unexpected, and to show up when and where it matters most.

References

Allshouse, C., Comeau, M., Rodgers, R., & Wells, N. (2018). Families of children with medical complexity: A view from the front lines. *Pediatrics, 141*(Suppl 3), S195–S201. https://doi.org/10.1542/peds.2017-1284D

American Board of Pediatrics. (2024, July 26). *Yearly growth in general pediatrics residents by demographics and program characteristics.* https://www.abp.org/dashboards/yearly-growth-general-pediatrics-residents-demographics-and-program-characteristics. Accessed January 22, 2025.

Ames, S. G., Delaney, R. K., Houtrow, A. J., Delgado-Corcoran, C., Alvey, J., Watt, M. H., & Murphy, N. (2023). Perceived disability-based discrimination in health care for children with medical complexity. *Pediatrics, 152*(1), e2022060975. https://doi.org/10.1542/peds.2022-060975

Anderson, H. L., Lewis, N., & Rezet, B. (2024). A qualitative study of resident advocacy work. *Pediatrics, 153*(3), e2023061590. https://doi.org/10.1542/peds.2023-061590

Bogetz, J. F., Bogetz, A. L., Bergman, D., Turner, T., Blankenburg, R., & Ballantine, A. (2014). Challenges and potential solutions to educating learners about pediatric complex care. *Academic Pediatrics, 14*(6), 603–609. https://doi.org/10.1016/j.acap.2014.06.004

Bogetz, J. F., Bogetz, A. L., Rassbach, C. E., Gabhart, J. M., & Blankenburg, R. L. (2015). Caring for children with medical complexity: Challenges and educational opportunities identified by pediatric residents. *Academic Pediatrics, 15*(6), 621–625. https://doi.org/10.1016/j.acap.2015.08.004

Cohen, E., Kuo, D. Z., Agrawal, R., Berry, J. G., Bhagat, S. K. M., Simon, T. D., & Srivastava, R. (2011). Children with medical complexity: An emerging population for clinical and research initiatives. *Pediatrics, 127*(3), 529–538. https://doi.org/10.1542/peds.2010-0910

Dall, T. M., Reynolds, R. L., Chakrabarti, R., Forte, G. J., Langelier, M., Wang, S., Whyte, J., Sridhara Ankam, N., Annaswamy, T. M., Fredericson, M., Jain, N. B., Perret Karimi, D., Morgenroth, D. C., Slocum, C., & Wisotzky, E. (2021). The physiatry workforce in 2019 and beyond, part 2: Modeling results. *American Journal of Physical Medicine & Rehabilitation, 100*(9), 877–884. https://doi.org/10.1097/PHM.0000000000001659

Foster, C., Lin, E., Feinstein, J. A., Seltzer, R., Graham, R. J., Coleman, C., Ward, E., Coller, R. J., Sobotka, S., & Berry, J. G. (2025). Home health care research for children with disability and medical complexity. *Pediatrics, 155*(2), e2024067966. https://doi.org/10.1542/peds.2024-067966

Goldshore, M. A., Solomon, B. S., Downs, S. M., Pan, R., & Minkovitz, C. S. (2014). Residency exposures and anticipated future involvement in community settings. *Academic Pediatrics, 14*(4), 341–347. https://doi.org/10.1016/j.acap.2014.02.011

Health Resources & Services Administration (HRSA) Maternal and Child Health Bureau. (2022). *Children and youth with special health care needs NSCH Data Brief, 2019-2020.* https://mchb.hrsa.gov/data-research/national-survey-childrens-health

Houlihan, B. V., Coleman, C., Kuo, D. Z., Plant, B., & Comeau, M. (2024). What families of children with medical complexity say they need: Humanism in care delivery change. *Pediatrics, 153*(Suppl 1), e2023063424F. https://doi.org/10.1542/peds.2023-063424F

Ligibel, J. A., Goularte, N., Berliner, J. I., Bird, S. B., Brazeau, C. M. L. R., Rowe, S. G., Stewart, M. T., & Trockel, M. T. (2023). Well-being parameters and intention to leave current institution among academic physicians. *JAMA Network Open, 6*(12), e2347894. https://doi.org/10.1001/jamanetworkopen.2023.47894

McClafferty, H. (2024). Workforce concerns: Professional self care, personal readiness, impact of the pandemic, and other factors that impact the workforce. *Pediatric Clinics of North America, 71*(3), 413–429. https://doi.org/10.1016/j.pcl.2024.03.001

McPherson, M., Arango, P., Fox, H., Lauver, C., McManus, M., Newacheck, P. W., Perrin, J. M., Shonkoff, J. P., & Strickland, B. (1998). A new definition of children with special health care needs. *Pediatrics, 102*(1), 137–140. https://doi.org/10.1542/peds.102.1.137

Murphy Salem, S., Chase, B., Newman, L. R., Cohen, A. P., Cheston, C., & Huth, K. (2022). Perspectives on complex care training in a large academic pediatric training program. *Academic Pediatrics, 22*(5), 867–872. https://doi.org/10.1016/j.acap.2022.03.008

Rushton, F. E., Jr., & American Academy of Pediatrics Committee on Community Health Services. (2005). The pediatrician's role in community pediatrics. *Pediatrics, 115*(4), 1092–1094. https://doi.org/10.1542/peds.2004-2680

Shanafelt, T. D. (2021). Physician well-being 2.0: Where are we and where are we going? *Mayo Clinic Proceedings, 96*(10), 2682–2693. https://doi.org/10.1016/j.mayocp.2021.06.005

Sieplinga, K., Kruger, C., & Goodwin, E. (2023). Is it too complex? A survey of pediatric residency program's educational approach for the care of children with medical complexity. *BMC Medical Education, 23*(1), 331. https://doi.org/10.1186/s12909-023-04324-y

Turk, M. A., Gans, B. M., Kim, H., & Alter, K. E. (2023). A call for action: Increasing the pediatric rehabilitation medicine workforce. *Journal of Pediatric Rehabilitation Medicine, 16*(3), 449–455. https://doi.org/10.3233/PRM-230044

Vinci, R. J. (2021). The pediatric workforce: Recent data trends, questions, and challenges for the future. *Pediatrics, 147*(6), e2020013292. https://doi.org/10.1542/peds.2020-013292

Yu, J. A., Bayer, N. D., Beach, S. R., Kuo, D. Z., & Houtrow, A. J. (2022). A national profile of families and caregivers of children with disabilities and/or medical complexity. *Academic Pediatrics, 22*(8), 1489–1498. https://doi.org/10.1016/j.acap.2022.08.004

Yu, J. A., McKernan, G., Hagerman, T., Schenker, Y., & Houtrow, A. (2021). Identifying children with medical complexity from the National Survey of Children's Health combined 2016-17 data set. *Hospital Pediatrics, 11*(2), 192–197. https://doi.org/10.1542/hpeds.2020-0180

Index

A
Ableism, 51, 62–63, 94
ACE Kids Act, 82–85
Advocacy, 22, 24, 33, 46, 51, 61, 91–97

C
Care, 1, 11, 39, 51, 69, 91
Care coordination, 13–15, 17, 18, 23–28, 72, 73, 76, 81, 93
Children with medical complexity (CMC), 1, 11, 39, 51, 70, 91
Chronic health conditions, 1, 41, 44, 51
Complex care pediatricians, 4, 12, 92, 94
Complex care programs, 4–5, 12–16, 18, 20, 71, 96
Coordination, 3, 17, 18, 23–27, 30, 73, 74, 77

D
Decision-making, 18, 19, 28, 29, 45, 52–55, 57–61, 63, 70, 79, 93
Disability rights, 51, 61–63, 97

F
Family caregivers, 43, 45, 94
Functional impairments, 2, 5

G
Goals of care, 21, 59
Guardianship, 29, 57–60

H
Healthcare costs, 2, 72
Healthcare payment models, 70, 76–81, 84–86
Healthcare systems, 1, 3, 11, 13, 14, 26, 27, 39, 44, 45, 59, 62, 63, 69, 78, 85, 86, 91–92, 96
Healthcare value, 73
Health policy, 3, 97
Home nursing, 19, 42–43
Humanism, 92

M
Medicaid waiver programs, 82, 83
Medical ethics, 52, 53, 55, 94, 97
Medical home, 3, 4, 7, 12–15, 17, 18, 23, 24, 39, 41, 73, 83–85, 96
Models of care, 4, 12, 15, 17, 23, 51, 73–76, 85

P
Parents as partners, 94, 95
Pediatric workforce, 12, 92–94
Public health, 3–5, 7, 22, 51, 52, 82, 91–97

S
Shared decision-making, 4, 16–18, 20–22, 32, 53, 55–56, 70, 93
Siblings of children with medical complexity, 40–42

Social determinants of health, 39–40, 74, 78, 94, 97
Special healthcare needs, 1, 11, 16, 40, 91

T
Transition to adult care, 60
Transitions to adulthoods, 27–33, 57–61

The manufacturer's authorised representative in the EU is Springer Nature Customer Service Centre GmbH, Europaplatz 3, 69115 Heidelberg, Germany. If you have any concerns regarding our products, please contact ProductSafety@springernature.com

Printed and bound by CPI Group (UK) Ltd, Croydon, CR0 4YY

26/03/2026

02078977-0003